CONTENTS

THE 30-DAY CARNIVORE MEAL PLAN

As with all dietary changes, please discuss your nutritional needs with a qualified healthcare professional.

The 30-Day Carnivore Meal Plan is more than a meal plan. It is your complete 30-day guide to transformation from a plant eater to a meat eater. During this month you will eat a more biologically-appropriate diet than you probably ever have in your life. Look out - your life will forever be changed.

As you use the 30-Day Carnivore Meal Plan you'll learn new cooking methods, and become a pro at making a perfect steak, roast, and burger every time. You'll experience the calm self-assured confidence that comes when you are eating at the top of the food chain. You'll feel how your body was meant to feel when it's eating foods that support optimal health.

You'll also experience some adjustments - whether it's as simple as having to supplement extra salt as your body learns to balance electrolytes in the new leaner, less-inflamed version of yourself or you experience a 'healing crisis' as your body processes out the oxalates, excess hormones stored in fat, and other toxins that have backed up in your system due to a lifetime of eating a sub-optimal diet.

This meal plan guides you through the ultimate elimination diet. The carnivore diet is used for extreme health conditions, as a nutrient-dense health reset, a weight-loss strategy, and/or as an experiment in human nutrition. This month we are going to see what our body does when eating only animal products!

The Carnivore Meal Plan is made up of distinct weeks that include different categories.

1. Meat and Salt
2. Meat, Salt, and Eggs
3. Meat, Salt, Eggs, and Dairy
4. Meat, Salt, Dairy, Eggs, and Seasonings

Most people will want to start in the 4th, least restrictive, category and then transition to a more strict version once they are feeling the benefits of increased mental clarity, energy, and stable mood that comes with the carnivore diet.

ABOUT CARA

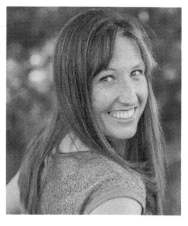

In February 2019 Cara Comini started the carnivore diet, in an effort to 'prove that the carnivore diet didn't work'. In reality, within 3 days she felt enormous benefits, most of all improving her lingering mental health issues.

Coming from an already healthy ketogenic diet, Cara was shocked at how the counterintuitive Carnivore diet worked so well for so many things ... from giving her more energy to clearing up minor skin issues, to increasing strength and endurance, improving sleep, and more.

Passionate to share, she put together this meal plan to take the guess-work out of the carnivore diet so that you can see if this way of eating works for you as well!

Cara Comini is a health skeptic and mother of 3. She writes at the blog Health Home and Happiness about natural living after seeing how dietary protocols make drastic changes in her own family's health. She has been using nutrition to lessen the symptoms of chronic conditions in her family since 2008 when she started using diet to treat autism in her daughter.

Cara enjoys being outside with her 3 children and resides in the mountains of Montana. They have a very eat-to-live philosophy, and prioritize healthy foods because it gives them the energy and good attitude to have fun outdoors. Family favorites include skiing, fishing, camping, hiking, and road trips.

Visit Health Home and Happiness on YouTube to see her personal updates, recipe videos, and samples of daily 'what I ate today' on the carnivore diet.

STARTING THE CARNIVORE DIET

The version of carnivore diet that you start with is completely personal preference. Take a look through the weekly menus to see what appeals to you, and then develop your own personal game plan.

Some people will find that eggs or dairy mess with their digestion, but including a limited amounts of seasonings and sauces works just fine for them. Others may find the opposite - meat, dairy, and eggs are all excellent but any introduction of seasonings or spices causes a digestion issue.

Everyone is individual, and the only way to know for sure is to experiment and see what works for you at this time.

If you dive in to the most strict version of the carnivore diet (just meat and salt) and find that a couple days (or hours!) in you are burning out, please remember that even a little amount of progress is better than what you're currently doing!

If being carnivore is your goal...

...it's better to include eggs than give up on the carnivore diet completely.

...it's better to include sauces and seasonings than give up on the carnivore diet completely.

....it's better to eat cheese than give up on the carnivore diet completely.

....if you know you're going to be going off carnivore for a meal, a day, or a week, it's better to treat yourself with keto-friendly foods than carb-laden foods.

If doing a zero-carb (carnivore) trial is your goal, and you're not quite making it, even if you cheat, aim for 'closer to carnivore than you ate last month' and you'll be headed in the right direction.

Don't let *your perfectionism* be the enemy of your progress.

That said, some of you are **complete rock stars** and you are going to start with the most strict version, white knuckle through the first couple days, and emerge triumphantly. If this is you, I admire your dedication, perseverance, and willpower, and I can't wait to seeing and hearing what results you get!

WHAT IS THE CARNIVORE DIET?

Carnivore, also called zero-carb, allows foods that come from animals only.

There are no 'carnivore police', and of course you are free to eat what you want to eat, but in general the carnivore diet will include:

• Meat from any animal, including organ meats and bone broth. Meat can be cooked in any way (Instant Pot, slow cooked, grilled, etc)
• Eggs from any animal including chicken, duck, goose, quail.
• Dairy, for some people, especially high fat dairy. Most people who do the carnivore diet also enjoy the benefits of being in ketosis and a diet where most of the calories come from fat. Dairy is naturally high in fat, and when it is aged (such as cheese) it is lower in carbohydrate. Favorites include: Butter, heavy whipping cream, cheese, and cultured cream.
• Honey, which some include on carnivore but nearly every recipe in this meal plan omits honey.
• Salt and other electrolytes (potassium, magnesium). Historically salt has been a prized commodity, and it is necessary for most people . who are starting out on the carnivore diet.

FOODS NOT INCLUDED IN THE CARNIVORE DIET:

Plants of any kind, including:
• Oils that come from plants including coconut, MCT, avocado, or olive oil.
• Fruit or vegetables in any form.
• Sweeteners, including stevia, or sugar - both are plants. In addition, artificial sweeteners, even etrythritol, are avoided to avoid the potential insulin response.

Note on animal foods, plant oils, and carbs: Though there are carbohydrates present in seafood, eggs, and cheese, they are still relatively low. You may hear 'carnivore' also called 'zero carb'. The term 'zero carb' refers to the old-fashioned food categories; meat and eggs were considered protein and plants were considered 'carbs'.

This gets confusing in relation to this diet and modern nutrition labeling as plant oils (soybean, canola, coconut) all do not have any carbs listed, but aren't part of the carnivore/zero carb diet. In contrast, scallops, eggs, and some dairy contain some carbohydrates but are included on a carnivore/zero-carb diet.

FOODS THAT ARE INCLUDED BY SOME ON CARNIVORE, BUT NOT PURISTS:

- Coffee or black or green tea, no sweetener.
- Herbs and spices to season meat.
- Sauces for flavor and texture, not necessarily nutrition: BBQ sauce, mayo, mustard, ketchup, etc.
- Condiments, especially fermented condiments like fermented pickle relish, sauerkraut, horseradish sauce.

WHAT TO BUY FOR
THE CARNIVORE DIET

See the grocery lists at the start of each weekly meal plan for an idea of what you will be eating for the week.

In addition to muscle meat, liver and seafood of some form is recommended weekly, or at least monthly due to the high nutrient density. We have a delicious Liver Pate recipe (page 52) that can be spread on steak or eaten with pork rinds for a 'chip and dip' meat treat included in this book.

Scallops, salmon, muscles, crab, and other seafood provide a taste and texture change, and are a good source of iodine and other nutrients.

Your specific budget and nutrient needs will dictate the quality of meat, eggs, and dairy that you get.

QUALITY CONSIDERATIONS

For those with the ability to, I recommend all grass fed/pastured meats and wild-caught seafood. Dairy ideally comes from cows feasting on grass, with minimal-to-no grain supplement.

For those who can't do all grass fed/wild caught, I recommend prioritizing seafood as wild-caught, and then as much grass fed beef and pork and fat as you can afford. *Beef and pork are more calorie-dense than lighter meat, so you'll get more calories for your dollar if you prioritize here.*

In my family we eat a lot of wild game (elk, venison) since we're hunters. I also get a delivery monthly of really good beef and pork from ButcherBox. See the resource page at thecarnivoremealplan.com for a discount code and how to get the most delicious meat for your money from Butcherbox. Then I fill in as we run out with 'grocery store' meat - beef, chicken, and some pork. Organ meat I get from a fantastic local butcher, but if you don't have a butcher that carries it, US Wellness Meats is a great source.

Liver and other offal such as marrow bones, heart, and tongue can often be found inexpensively even from grassfed organic animals. Epic and a few other brands have grassfed tallow on Amazon, which again, are very inexpensive calorie-wise!

If the budget is tight, do not be put off if you have to buy all your meat from the grocery store and skip the organic! Meat, eggs, and dairy without additives are still incredibly nutrient-dense foods.

CONVENTIONAL MEATS, ETHICS, ANIMAL NUTRITION

There are some ranches that are awful, and you may have seen some of these highlighted in documentaries. But in general, and living in Montana I know more than my fair share of them, farmers and ranchers really take care of their animals well.

Nearly all beef cattle are pastured for the vast majority of their diet because they are raised where there is a lot of pasture, and it keeps the cattle healthy and it's free! The difference between conventional beef (what is in most grocery stores) and grassfed/organic is that the conventional beef is supplemented with grain and soy to bring the weight up faster.* This is a supplement, not their only food. Ranchers know that stressed cattle make poor meat, and they take great care of their cattle, whether they are finishing them on grass or supplementing with grain and soy.

Every calving season (which often occurs when it's still snowy) ranchers drop everything they are doing to help the cows. My sister-in-law is a 'ranch wife' in Nebraska, and every calving season I get pictures by text of calves that she's been instructed to 'keep alive' that are wrapped in old towels and blankets, being bottle fed, and taking up residence in her laundry room until snows or floods pass, or they become strong enough to make it on their own. I feel like ranchers that supplement with grain get a bad reputation among the health-conscious crowd, and I'd like to reiterate that the vast majority of ranchers absolutely bend over backwards to help these cows have a good quality of life.

SELECTING MEAT AT THE GROCERY STORE FOR COST SAVINGS

When you select meat at the grocery store, make it a habit to cruise the meat department on a regular basis and learn when they mark down their meat. Meat that is marked down for quick sale can be stocked up on by freezing. Just use it the same day you thaw it, and it is perfectly healthy to consume!

Get to know your prices, and if price is an issue, ground beef, roasts, and pork are going to be on your plate often. Enjoy them! We have numerous recipes for roasts to make them delicious and tender in this book.

Other less-expensive high-nutrition cuts of meat include liver, stock bones and bone marrow, heart, and tongue, and if you look around you may find them available at a local grocery store or inexpensive from a local butcher.

It is also possible to find natural all-meat hot dogs now, which makes a great quick meal.

> *Why does pastured (grass fed) meat cost so much more?*
>
> *When cows are completely grass fed/grass finished, it takes them double the amount of time to get up to their slaughter weight. This extra time means extra work and care for the ranchers, which is why grass fed/finished beef costs more than grain-fed. Also, the corn/soy fed to conventional cattle to fatten them up are produced with lots of government subsidies, so the grain fed to cattle is artificially low in cost, which creates a somewhat misleading price in the grocery store.*

PERSONAL CARE PRODUCTS ON CARNIVORE:

When going carnivore, you may wonder about personal care products like shampoo, lotion, and deodorant. These products have become more and more toxic and are a common source of carcinogens, endocrine disruption (which can cause tumors, hormone imbalances, infertility, developmental delay, and more), and a general increase in the toxic load that the gut, kidneys, and liver have to process.

Because they are not ingested, personal care products are not as important as what we are eating. Still, some of them will be absorbed through our skin. *Avoiding chemicals as much as possible is helpful for returning the body to its natural toxin-eliminating nutrient-processing state.*

Do your body, digestion, and mind a favor by taking a break from the toxic load present in conventional personal care products. This doesn't have to be forever, but as you start making healthy changes, allow your body to get maximum benefit of this increased nutrition by reducing your toxic load as much as possible.

Tallow makes amazing personal care products. Tallow balm is an excellent moisturizer, and you can get it scented or unscented. Tallow soap is a traditional soap, and though hard to find, it does exist! See the Carnivore Resource Page for recommendations.

Carnivore shampoo: You can wash your hair with egg yolk! To use this carnivore-friendly 'shampoo' Carefully separate the yolk from the white, and then use 1 yolk as shampoo. This works best with warm, not hot, water.

Essential oils can be used as desired - again, personal care is a personal choice and there are no hard or fast carnivore rules here.

For makeup, sunscreen, skincare, and shaving needs for you men, I highly recommend BeautyCounter for safer skincare products! You can find a link on the Carnivore Resource Page to my recommended products.

De-stink while reducing your toxic load: there are lots of natural deodorants out there. A simple option is to spray with Everclear (the alcohol). This will kill bacteria and may be enough odor protection for some. For others, Schmidt's, Native, or Primal Pit Paste are natural alternatives to conventional stick deodorant.

On the topic of deodorant... When you first go into ketosis, which will happen with the carnivore diet, your body makes tons and tons of ketones. For the first 4-6 weeks you may find that you s.t.i.n.k. as one of the byproducts of making ketones is an acetone-like substance. As you become fat adapted, you'll start producing just as many ketones as you need.

Until you become fat adapted, though, drinking extra water can get your body to dump those strong-smelling byproducts into your urine rather than having them excrete out your sweat glands.

HOW TO TRANSITION ONTO THE CARNIVORE DIET

THE CARNIVORE DIET FROM A CARBOHYDRATE-BASED DIET

The majority of people in industrialized countries are carbohydrate-based. This means that they get most of their energy and power their brain with glucose, which they derive from carbohydrates.

If you follow one of these diets, your transition to carnivore takes an extra step to be less difficult. We'll talk about that in a minute.

- Standard American diet, whether you're following the food pyramid or eating the 'standard' of way too much junk food.
- Paleo or primal diets, if you are including fruit, honey, and/or sweet potatoes.
- Gluten-free diet
- Dairy-free diet
- Vegetarian and vegan diets
- Any other diet that includes at least one serving of fruit, sugar or natural sweetener, or grains each day.

You will see shocking benefits on keto - and it gets even BETTER on carnivore - it's quite amazing what changing your diet can do for your health - both physical and mental!

If you are a 'carb burner' and currently eating more than 30ish grams of carbohydrate a day, you can decide between these two options for starting the carnivore diet:

1. Go immediately on the carnivore diet, and deal with a rough 6 weeks but at the end of the 6 weeks you'll be fully adapted to carnivore and will probably have lost a bunch of weight (if desired) and feel amazing.

Or

2. Become fat adapted first by first transitioning onto the ketogenic (keto) diet for 4-6 weeks, and then starting the carnivore diet from there.

If you choose to start carnivore right away, all you need to do is eat all animal foods and no plant foods, as is outlined in this book, and wait out the roller coaster of your body adjusting over the next 6 weeks.

If you choose to start keto first, learn the keto diet and give yourself a month of meat-heavy keto to adjust to ketosis using a whole-foods, meat-heavy keto approach.

For help transitioning onto keto, see the resources page that goes with this book at thecarnivoremealplan.com

THE CARNIVORE DIET FROM KETO

Many people come to the carnivore diet from the keto diet - meaning their body is already in ketosis and fat adapted. The transition to carnivore is much easier if you are already fat adapted.

Fat adaption (also called keto adapted) is the state of being adapted to using ketones as fuel.

Signs of being fat adapted are:

- Showing less ketones in your urine on ketone strips.
- Having more endurance during exercise.
- Being able to skip a meal without excessive hunger or lightneadedness.

Because you are already adapted to being in ketosis, and with keto you likely have slowed (or completely stopped!) your cravings of carbohydrates and reduced some inflammation already, the transition onto carnivore is relatively simple and easy.

> *If you haven't yet adjusted to being in ketosis, you may get the keto flu. This is covered more in depth in the Keto Family Class (See resource page).*
>
> *If you're new to eating keto or low-carb, the Keto Family Class will get you into ketosis in as little as 24 hours, using family-friendly keto foods that are delicious and simple to prepare. The Keto Family Class contains everything that you need to get from sugar/carb burning to fat adapted in under 2 months.*

There are still four considerations that you'll want to take as you transition onto the carnivore diet from a keto diet:

1. Inflammation down = salt needs up temporarily.

When you stop eating food that irritates your body, your body stops having a constant inflammatory response. This results in a couple pounds of weight loss (usually) just like when you started keto - and this time it's from inflammation.

With this water weight loss, the body needs to adjust again to having less water weight to dissolve the salt in. Usually this adjustment takes 30 days, but until those 30 days are up your needs for salt may be much more than you're used to - even on keto.

To remedy this electrolyte imbalance take 1/4 teaspoon of sea salt followed by a tall glass of water (warm or cold) 3-4 times a day or whenever you feel tired or dehydrated.

2. Your appreciation, and connection with your food will change. Meat is your fuel, and we're taking the quick hit that comes with eating keto treats that you may have been consuming.

You may think of meat as boring now, but when that's all you're eating, you come to deeply appreciate it! Different cuts, methods of cooking, textures, and how salty the meat is provides more variety than you may realize. From silky smooth bone broth, to tender slow-cooked brisket, chilled cooked shrimp, creamy liver pate, crisp bacon, baked chicken with flakey salty skin, and of course the ever-popular fatty ribeye provide the nutrients and variety you need.

3. You will probably need to eat more meat than you currently are, but within reason.

Duh, right?

You also need to plan to replace everything that you have been eating with meat! Some of us have had it drilled into our heads that we only need to eat a couple servings of meat each day - and servings should be the size and shape of the palm of our hand.

If you only eat this much meat, you're going to be hungry! Most people on the carnivore diet will eat 1-2 pounds of meat a day. Red meat with extra fat added will provide the most calories, but for flavor, texture, and micro nutrient variety you can add in other kinds of meat as well.

While counting calories isn't a required part of the carnivore diet, if you're hungry, feeling low energy, or overall not feeling fantastic - do a spot check with a calorie counting app or by looking up nutrition facts of the amount of meat you eat in a day. If you're under 1500 (or whatever your personal calorie needs are), most of the time that will explain why you're not feeling well!

On the other end of the spectrum, most people will not need to gorge themselves on meat every day in order to feel well on the carnivore diet. Unless you are abnormally tall, muscular, or active, the same 1-2 pounds of meat is probably plenty! Some body builders or competitive athletes highlight that they stay trim and fit on 3+ pounds of meat a day, but these people are outliers

Remember, calories aren't the be-all end-all of eating well, but they are a useful tool to gauge how much you should be eating.

3. Your body may go into rapid repair mode at the start of this diet.

If you are tired the first few weeks on carnivore, rejoice!

Wait? What?!

This excessive tiredness is because your body is healing. Your energy will come, and your light will shine brighter than ever when your body has done its thing with the nutrients and rest you are providing for it. If you get a boost of energy from carnivore, you may be doing a 'slow and steady' repair, or not have that much wrong to begin with.

One more consideration, that we're not going to elaborate on here because it's not a problem for most people, is that you may 'dump oxalates'. If you notice skin rashes, joint pain, or digestive trouble it may oxalate dumping. In that case, do a search and learn about managing oxalates - it just means you need to add some back in for a time and then taper off to reduce the dumping.

HOW TO USE THIS MEAL PLAN AND WHAT TO EXPECT THE FIRST WEEK OR TWO

This 30-Day Carnivore Meal Plan provides different breakfast, lunch, and dinner recipes. These are just suggestions, and not essential to doing the carnivore diet! See the next chapter on intermittent fasting if eating less than 3 times a day sounds appealing to you.

Carnivore is a good exercise in using food as fuel, and breaking the habit of using food for reward or comfort or even a creative outlet.

CHOOSE YOUR VERSION OF CARNIVORE

Looking through this meal plan, you will notice there are multiple versions of the carnivore diet. The 'most true' version is just meat and salt and water. But many people find success (and ease of compliance) with the most liberal version of meat, dairy, eggs, and seasonings! Each meal plan will guide you through a sample week of eating.

After that week, you can either choose a different (more or less restrictive) week from the meal plan to follow, repeat the same week again, or repeat your favorite recipes and add in others that you will enjoy.

CALORIE TRACKING

You may find that some days you are very hungry, and some days you are barely hungry at all. If you are doing this for weight loss or weight gain, you'll probably want to track your calories. But if not, feel free to just listen to your body's cues and eat as desired.

On each page of this meal plan, calories are listed as well as overall fat/protein percentages. This helps you know whether you feel better eating more fat, more protein, or an even mix.

TIME SPENT COOKING

By going carnivore you may also **free up an hour or more a day** that you had previously spent selecting and shopping for and preparing meals.

Just think... what will you do with your extra hour a day?

The carnivore diet is the ultimate minimalist diet. You can get creative while using meat if you desire, but at its most simple form- frying up a steak and maybe an egg or two in a cast iron skillet is a shocking break from over-complicated nutrient-inferior recipes that you may be currently cooking on a daily basis.

FEELING STRONGER AND MORE CLEAR

During the first weeks of carnivore, you will notice your head clear, depression and anxiety start to lift, and you just feel overall better. You will find a new motivation to pick heavy things up and move them around.

Your confidence will uptick, and you will feel the calm assurance that you would expect comes from being at the top of the food chain.

Check in with your body and mind throughout your carnivore experience, and note how you feel differently from day to day.

Even if you are only doing a month-long carnivore challenge, the experience is sure to be life changing.

FASTING AND THE CARNIVORE DIET

Fasting is not necessary on the carnivore diet, but some form of fasting is often incorporated. Many people find that it is easier to stick with the carnivore diet if they eat just once or twice a day, and fast the rest of the day, also called 'intermittent fasting'.

TO INCORPORATE INTERMITTENT FASTING WITH THIS MEAL PLAN:

Choose to cook all the food suggestions at once for one big 'feast' meal, or you can double or triple whatever meal sounds the best to you and eat enough to meet your nutrients needs. With the nutrition information on each recipe provided, it's easy to see at a glance how much food you should make for your one or two meals a day.

WHAT IS FASTING?

Fasting is a simple concept, but also foreign in our age of eat-eat-eat. Fasting is abstaining from calories for a set period of time. Usually, non-calorie beverages such as black coffee and tea, and water are allowed but no food is.

Salt and other electrolytes are included in extended fasts (24 hours or longer)

Fasting allows your body a break from constant digestion, and gives it time to do other things - like clean up old cells, balance hormones, and even build muscle!

To learn more about how fasting works, including safety precautions for extended fasting and how to break a fast, The Complete Guide To Fasting by Dr. Jason Fung and Jimmy Moore is an excellent science-backed guide to fasting. .

THE BENEFITS OF FASTING

Fasting is an ancient practice and, despite what the companies who sell you snack foods want you to believe, is very good for us!

Some of the benefits of fasting include:

- Increased blood glucose control.
- Easier calorie and weight management.
- Better performance during fasted exercise.
- Clearer thinking and more focus mentally.
- Tracking calories, if needed, becomes simpler.
- Simplicity of only needing to eat once or twice a day.
- Increased growth hormone, which leads to increased lean body mass (muscle) and decreased fat accumulation.

HUNGER HORMONES

Just like sleeping is tied to hormones, your hunger is tied to hormones. When you understand this, you understand that just like having a consistent sleep schedule can make it easier to sleep when you're supposed to sleep and be awake when you're supposed to be awake you can do the same thing with hunger!

Being hungry isn't an emergency* - you may have been conditioned to think that once you're hungry, you have to eat or you'll just keep getting more hungry. That isn't true. If you want to start fasting, you'll find that you get hungry around the times that you typically eat, and then after that time has passed, you no longer feel hungry.

If you're 'always hungry' and eat all day long, it's likely that you've just trained your body to expect food all day long. You can re-train your body to eat less often by shifting when and how often you eat.

Of course, other things can come into play with hunger - if your body really is requiring more energy due to increased exercise, recovery from an illness or injury, nutrient demands from pregnancy or breastfeeding or growth in children, it will send out hunger signals despite your desire to eat less often.

If you find you are extra hungry at a particular day - go ahead and eat extra! But if you're always hungry all the time, that's a good indication that your hunger hormones have been trained to be secreted at all time, and you will benefit from reigning them in with intermittent fasting.

*Insulin resistance can cause hunger to become a hypoglycmic issue. This can be corrected primarily by eating a lower-carbohydrate diet like carnivore! For more information on insulin resistance and how carnivore helps see page 103.

INTERMITTENT FASTING

Intermittent fasting is any fast that is intentional and is less than 24 hours. The most common acronyms for fasting are expressed like this: 16:8, 20:4, and OMAD.

Technically everyone practices intermittent fasting. Fasting is any period that you are not eating, so we all fast as we sleep. Intermittent fasting as discussed here means intentionally fasting for set periods of time that are longer than we may be used to.

Eating windows: When you intermittent fast, you have defined hours for eating and defined hours for fasting. These hours are expressed as numbers such as 16:8 or 20:4 and refer to the time of the day you're fasting, and the time of the day you're eating.

So if you have a 16:8 schedule then you fast for 16 hours out of the 24-hour day and eat during a an 8-hour block. Your 'eating window' refers to the hours that you are eating. An eating window in a 16:8 schedule may be from 8:00 a.m. to 4:00 p.m. if you prefer to eat early, or 11:00 a.m. to 7:00 p.m. if you prefer to eat later - or any other set 8-hour block.

OMAD means One Meal A Day. People who eat OMAD eat all their food in one sitting, usually within a 1-hour time period.

If you haven't noticed yet, intermittent fasting is really just an overly-complex way of saying you 'skip breakfast'. or 'skip dinner'. Some people like the detailed explanation, and to understand all the terminology used in online discussion groups, but it's really not complicated at all.

EXTENDED FASTING

Extended fasting refers to any fast that is over 24 hours. Yes, this is safe! If you are in the habit of overeating, and need to do a reset, a 24-48-hour fast may be exactly what you need.

Some health organizations promote a yearly or every-6-month period of fasting for 5-7 days to boost health and give the body a break. There are some important considerations to take when breaking (ending) an extended fast, which are not covered here. Seek the advice from a professional, whether in person or by a book, before attempting an extended fast beyond 72-hours.

WATER FASTING

Water fasting is the most common type of fasting, whether it is an extended fast or intermittent fast.

Some advocate that only filtered water should be consumed during a water fast. Others include any non-sweet no-calorie beverage into a 'water fast' including black coffee, tea, and even flavored (but not sweetened) seltzer water.

Avoiding sweeteners, even natural sweeteners like stevia, is recommended during a water fast as sweeteners can affect hormones in some people and negate some of the benefits of fasting.

DRY FASTING

Dry fasting is less common and it includes going without food or liquid for a certain amount of time. Dry fasting is said to promote the autophagy part of fasting more than water fasting, and is usually done for a shorter amount of time. Obviously dehydration could be a concern, so be sure to research dry fasting before attempting.

IF YOU CAN'T FAST

Fasting is by no means required to eat a carnivore diet! The main advice for carnivore is to eat when you are hungry, don't eat when you're not. You may find that you settle into a pattern of eating two smallish meals a day for 3-4 days and then eating 3 large meals for a couple days. This is just fine!

What you don't want to do, though, is eat little bits all day long. This puts your body in the constant state of digestion. Try to limit your eating window to 3 distinct meals so there is a definite start and stop to eating and not grazing all day.

This 3 or less meals-a-day goal will help you eat more balanced intentional meals rather than always having food in your mouth out of habit. It will also force you into other coping skills for boredom, sadness, fear, etc.

VERSIONS OF THE CARNIVORE DIET

Whether you are eating just meat and salt, or including everything from meat to dairy to eggs and even some seasonings, we detail what different versions of the carnivore diet include in this chapter.

MEAT AND SALT

This version of the carnivore diet includes meat, salt, water, and that is it. Supplementation with magnesium and potassium is also often helpful. Black coffee and black or green tea can be included if desired. Purists will avoid coffee and tea as well.

Fat is encouraged because when we avoid carbohydrates, the majority of our energy comes from fat. People typically find they feel best when getting at least 70% of their calories from fat, rather than the majority of their calories from protein. Individual needs and preferences may vary.

Salt is used to season, but even black pepper and herbs are avoided. Some autoimmune conditions are sensitive to spices including black pepper, so we really are giving our bodies a break.

Foods eaten when eating that the Meat & Salt version of the carnivore diet:

- Beef, especially fatty cuts
- Chicken, skin on and mostly dark meat for the best satiety
- Lamb
- Seafood including wild-caught shellfish
- Fish, especially fatty fish like salmon
- Pork if desired - some will want to avoid as pork can be hard for some people to digest.
- Meat stock or bone broth made with bones, marrow blended in or eaten separately.
- Organ meat including liver, kidney, sweetbreads, heart, fish eggs, and more from any animal.
- Any other uncured unseasoned meat including pork rinds seasoned only with sea salt, or jerky made with just sea salt and meat.
- Sea Salt

Some people will feel best still abstaining from eggs and/or dairy but including specific seasonings like pepper, garlic, and cinnamon with their meat. Dairy and eggs are common food allergies and/or intolerances, especially with those prone to seasonal allergies and/or skin rashes including eczema and psoriasis.

MEAT AND EGGS

The Meat and Eggs version of the carnivore diet includes meat, eggs, and salt, and that is it. As with just meat and salt, supplementation with magnesium and potassium is often helpful.

When eating meat and eggs, you want to make sure your eggs are *just eggs* from a shell. Scrambled eggs from restaurants or from a carton often have fillers such as wheat, soybean oil, and cellulose fiber. The problem with these fillers is that those fillers can cause inflammation or contain excess carbs and may make you think that you're having trouble with eggs, when in reality it's just the fillers that you're reacting to.

In this version of the carnivore diet, you can have everything under Meat & Salt plus:

• Eggs of any kind, including chicken, turkey, duck, etc.
• Raw egg yolks. Raw whites can be consumed, but they contain an anti-nutrient that binds to biotin, a B vitamin, so raw egg whites should be limited. Most of the nutrition from eggs are in the yolks anyway.

MEAT, EGGS, AND DAIRY

Dairy is a game-changer when you are on the carnivore diet. Creamy cream cheese, tangy yogurt and sour cream, melty cheddar, and heavy cream all add richness, flavor, and variety to carnivore. Kefir, cultured cream, and yogurt can all add probiotics as well.

Why wouldn't you include dairy in carnivore? Many people have a sensitivity or allergy to dairy. In addition, the mild creamy goodness of dairy makes it easy to over-eat, a problem with those who are doing carnivore for weight loss.

On the carnivore diet it is generally encouraged to use dairy as a condiment, not the main course. Mostly meat is the theme of most people's best version of the carnivore diet.

Foods included in addition to meat and eggs included:

• Homemade probiotic sour cream
• Commercial plain yogurt
• Milk kefir, plain (see the carnivore resource page for cultures)
• Cheese, store bought or homemade
• Colostrum
• Fluid milk, raw preferred
• Ghee and butter
• Heavy cream in coffee or tea

MEAT, DAIRY, EGGS, AND SEASONINGS (MOSTLY MEAT)

This version of carnivore includes meat, eggs, and salt, and also additional foods for flavor and texture, not for nutrition. Herbs may also be used as supplements.

This version of carnivore does have loads of benefits and is many people's best version of the carnivore diet because it:

- Keeps insulin low, which reduces hunger, promotes a healthy weight, and many more benefits.
- Keeps blood glucose stable, without big highs and lows.
- Provides variety and seasonings. If you grew up eating heavily seasoned foods, you may find spices harder to give up than sugar! In this version you can keep them in.
- Makes going out to eat easier. Without having to inspect every ingredient in every food, you can just choose meat, dairy, and eggs from the menu or when eating as a guest without having to cart your own plain meat-and-salt everywhere.

This version of carnivore represents the most liberal version of the carnivore diet, and is a great entry to carnivore. Many people find that a 'mostly meat' version of carnivore, that still includes other zero-carb foods as indicated here is the easiest version of the carnivore diet for them to stick with.

Others find that this version is not restrictive enough and opt to eliminate some or all seasonings.

Common seasonings and sauces to eliminate:
- Sugar in all forms
- Nightshades
- Black pepper
- Food additives
- Vegetable oils of any kind (mayo, marinades).

Foods included in addition to meat, dairy, and egg on the Meat, Dairy, Eggs, and Seasonings version of the Carnivore Diet:

- Herbs for flavor such as basil, chives, garlic, etc
- Spices such as black pepper, turmeric, cinnamon, and ginger
- Sauces as desired: Mayo, ketchup, mustard, BBQ sauce, etc.

MOSTLY MEAT KETO

Depending on who you talk to, this version is not technically carnivore. Mostly meat keto is one of the best ways to do the keto diet without getting sucked into the 'keto junk food' trap. Mostly meat keto is also a great way to transition to carnivore, whether you're coming from keto, the standard American diet, or something in between.

Mostly meat keto, as with most versions of carnivore, has most of your calories coming from animal products. However, plant foods are still used as condiments, and sometimes side dishes.

Mostly meat keto contains meat (or eggs) as your main dish, but you may also include a small side of green vegetables, a sprinkle here and there of nuts, caramelized onions on your burgers, sauerkraut and pickles, etc.

This version of keto makes it very easy to stay under 20-30 g of carb a day, with most people logging in well under 15 g of carbohydrate a day when they stick with eating mostly meat keto-friendly meals.

CARNIVORE   MEAT & SALT

SUNDAY

- **B** SALTED STOCK
- **L** CHICKEN THIGHS
- **D** BRISKET ROAST

MONDAY

- **B** RIBEYE
- **L** SCALLOPS
- **D** STOCK & LEFTOVER CHICKEN

TUESDAY

- **B** GRILLED SALMON
- **L** BRISKET AND TALLOW
- **D** MEATBALLS AND TALLOW

WEDNESDAY

- **B** LAMB CHOPS
- **L** BRISKET
- **D** MEATBALLS AND STOCK

THURSDAY

- **B** INSTANT POT HEART
- **L** BEEF SOUP
- **D** LIVER AND GROUND BEEF BURGERS, SHRIMP

FRIDAY

- **B** PORK SAUSAGE
- **L** BEEF SOUP
- **D** RIBS

SATURDAY

- **B** SALTED STOCK & PORK SAUSAGE
- **L** LEFTOVER RIBS
- **D** LEFTOVER BRISKET OR BEEF ROAST

MEAL PLAN

GROCERY List

MEAT

- ☐ Beef Marrow Bones or Osso Bucco, 2-3 lbs
- ☐ Brisket Roast, 4 lbs
- ☐ Ribeye, 8 ounces
- ☐ Ground Beef, 2-1/2 lbs *(additional 2 lbs for optional jerky)*
- ☐ *Beef, chuck roast (optional), 3 lbs*
- ☐ Chicken Thighs, skin on, 6
- ☐ Scallops, 1/2 lb
- ☐ Salmon, fillet, 6 oz
- ☐ Tallow, 1 pint
- ☐ Lamb Chops, 8 oz
- ☐ Beef Heart, 3-4 lbs
- ☐ Pork Rinds, 1 oz
- ☐ Liver, beef or chicken, 1 oz+
- ☐ Short Ribs, beef, 2 lbs
- ☐ Pork, ground, 1 lb

PANTRY

- ☐ Sea Salt
- ☐ *Optional Seasonings, see notes in recipe pages*

Salted Beef Stock

Sipping on stock (also called broth) can fill your need for electrolytes, take the place of other drinks, as well as provide inexpensive and easy-to-digest amino acids used for repair throughout the body.

2-3 pounds marrow bones or osso bucco + bones reserved from previous meals

1 tablespoon sea salt, or to taste

Instant Pot: Turn your Instant Pot to Saute - and adjust temperature control to medium. Allow pot to preheat for a minute or two, and then add your marrow bones. Do not use the lid for this step. Allow meat/bones to brown for 10-15 minutes and then turn. Turn Instant Pot off. Fill to the 'max' line on the stainless steel pot with filtered water.

Place lid on and adjust valve to 'seal'. Set Instant Pot to Pressure Cook, 90 minutes. After cooking, allow pressure to release naturally, this can take up to 30 minutes.

Slow cooker: Optionally, sear bones on the stove top over high heat or broil them for 5 minutes. Place bones in the bottom of the slow cooker and cover with filtered water until the slow cooker is 3/4 full. Cook on low for 8-24 hours.

Either method: Allow stock to cool a bit, so it is not so dangerous to pour. Remove meat, bones, and cartilage (save for another batch of stock or eat). Add salt and add the marrow and fat back in, pureeing with an immersion blender if desired.

Pour stock into jars using a funnel. Store stock in the refrigerator for up to 3 weeks.

Nutrition is approximate and will depend on the amount of meat and fat on your bones.

Nutrition per cup (approximate, including the marrow):
100 calories, 6 fat, 0 carb, 10 g protein

Chicken Thighs

1 tablespoon tallow or other fat, softened

6 chicken thighs, skin on

1 teaspoon sea salt

Preheat oven to 375* F.

Grease the bottom of a casserole dish that will fit the chicken thighs (8.5 x 11 works well) with fat. Place chicken thighs on top of the fat and sprinkle with sea salt.

Bake for 25-35 minutes, or until juices run clear. Enjoy!

Reserve half the chicken thighs for Monday.

Nutrition for 1/2 of recipe (3 chicken thighs):
899 calories, 55 fat, 2 carb, 101 g protein

SEASONING SUGGESTIONS:
Not everyone uses the carnivore diet as a complete elimination diet. If you wish to season with more than salt, here are seasoning suggestions.

Beef Stock: Add a few cloves of garlic, peeled and an inch of ginger, peeled, as well as 1 teaspoon of whole black peppercorns with the water. Strain out before eating.

Chicken: Zest a lemon and sprinkle over the skin, along with freshly-ground black pepper.

Brisket: Mix 1/4 cup sugar-free ketchup and 1 tablespoon apple cider vinegar and coat the roast before cooking, also using the salt as directed..

Brisket Roast

A full brisket is 8-20 pounds and will feed a crowd. For this week, so we don't get sick of brisket, we cook a portion of 4 pounds, yielding approx 3.5 pounds of cooked meat.

4-pound cut of brisket

1 tablespoon coarse sea salt or 1 teaspoon fine

1 cup filtered water if using Instant Pot

Instant Pot:
Sprinkle brisket with sea salt on all sides. Pour filtered water in the pot of the Instant Pot.
Place brisket fat-cap up in the Instant Pot, cutting into large pieces and stacking (keeping fat up on all pieces) if needed.
Cook at high pressure (manual) for 90 minutes and allow pressure to release naturally for at least 20 minutes, then use quick release to release the rest of the pressure.

Slow Cooker:
Sprinkle brisket with sea salt on all sides. Place fat-cap up in the slow cooker on its own (no water) and cook on low for 6-8 hours. Brisket is done when the meat around the edges is starting to be able to be shredded, but the whole roast doesn't fall apart when you pick it up with tongs.

Continue for either way of cooking:

Allow to rest for 10 minutes on the cutting board before slicing. Allow cooking liquid to set, and skim fat to use in cooking or add all the liquid to your beef stock
Cut across the grain into thin slices and top with tallow and salt if desired.

Makes 3.5 pounds cooked brisket; 7 servings of 8 ounces each.

MIND YOUR SALT!
It's common during the first 30-90 days of the carnivore diet to need to eat more salt than usual, even if you've previously been on keto. If you're feeling sluggish, or dehydrated, see how you feel after eating 1/4 teaspoon salt (plain) and then chugging a big glass of water. 9/10 times you'll feel much better within 10 minutes!

If salt doesn't help, you may be low in potassium or magnesium. Potassium chloride is a common salt substitute, called Low Salt or No Salt and can be used as salt, above, to supplement potassium. Magnesium citrate can also be supplemented as needed, or soaking in epsom salts (1 cup in the bath tub, filled to any amount, soaking for at least 10 minutes) can provide needed magnesium as well.

Nutrition per 8 ounces cooked brisket:
626 calories, 50 fat, 0 carb, 40 g protein

Ribeye

Starting the day with a rib eye is sure to satisfy! Don't be surprised if you're not hungry until well after your normal lunch time! See alternate ways to cook steak on page 31.

1 tablespoon tallow
8 ounce Ribeye
Sea Salt to taste

Cast Iron Pan Method

Preheat cast iron pan to medium high heat - if you're not sure, go higher. Preheat for at least 5 minutes. Pat your steak dry, and then salt the meat on both sides as the pan preheats.

Place steak on the in the pan and sear for 4 minutes.

Flip the steak using a thin metal spatula, and once flipped, immediately turn the heat to medium-low (3 on a scale of 1-10).

Cook an additional 10 minutes for a 3/4 to 1" steak, or until the edges of the steak start to feel like cartilage (like your nose, ear). Remember the steak will continue to cook as it rests. If in doubt, take it off early- you can always put it back on.

Remove the steak to a platter and allow to rest for 5 minutes before cutting. When cutting, using a sharp knife and slice against the grain.

> Nutrition: 8 oz ribeye and 1 teaspoon tallow:
> 696 calories, 56 g fat, 0 g carb, 48 g protein

Sea Scallops

Sea Scallops are sweet compared to other meat, and their creamy richness can satisfy a dessert craving like no other!

1/2 pound sea scallops

1 tablespoon tallow

Sea Salt

Rinse sea scallops and pat dry with a paper towel. Sprinkle with sea salt. Heat a skillet over medium-high heat and once the skillet is preheated, melt tallow. Tilt pan to cover with melted tallow.

Gently, being careful not to splash the hot tallow, place sea scallops in the pan and sear 1-2 minutes for small scallops, 2-3 minutes for large scallops.

Once seared, the scallops should lift up easily from the pan and be golden on the underside. Flip and then immediately reduce heat to medium-low and cook an additional 1-2 minutes for small and 2-3 minutes for large scallops.

Serve warm, sprinkling with more salt if desired.

> Nutrition for 1/2 pound of scallops + 1 tablespoon tallow:
> 315 calories, 15 fat, 6 carb, 34 g protein

Stock and Leftover Chicken

Bone-in skin on chicken is good cold, but you can also microwave or quickly heat it up in a greased skillet (covered) over medium heat.

2 chicken thighs, leftover from yesterday

2 cups salted beef stock

Reheating chicken options: In a pan over medium heat, skin side down, covered for 10 minutes. Or microwave for 45-90 seconds.

Reheat stock in a saucepan or microwave. You can also combine cubed chicken and stock and make a soup that you simmer in a saucepan.

Nutrition for 2 chicken thighs and 2 cups homemade broth: 632 calories, 38 fat, 0 carb, 70 g protein

SERVING SIZES:

Servings in this meal plan are designed to be 1500-1700 calories/day. Need more? Double or increase recipes as needed, and/or add extra fat.

In the Day Total box below you can see the fat percentages for each day. On just meat and salt it is typically higher in protein and lower in fat than the other versions of carnivore - if you feel better consuming more fat, but still want to stay 'meat and salt' find success by adding spoonfuls of tallow or other clarified animal fat on top of their meat with each meal.

Some people also will be able to add ghee (clarified butter) to their meat for extra fats and calories and deliciousness without problem.

Day Total:
1643 calories, 6 g carb, 109 g fat, 152 g protein.
1% carb, 38% protein, 61 % fat

On Monday we talked about pan-frying steaks on the stove top. There are other ways to cook steak, using more specialty tools.

GRILL

Preheat grill to medium high heat: 400* F or where you can only hold your hand 3" above the grill for 2-4 seconds. As you wait for the grill to preheat (approx 5-10 mins, depending on outside temp) salt the meat on both sides.

Place steak on the grill, and grill for 4-6 minutes. The key thing to watch for is the red liquid (myoglobin) will start to push up through the top of the meat. This is when it's time to flip for medium-well.

Flip, and again watch for the myoglobin to push up through the top of the meat. The second side usually takes a few minutes less than the first to cook.

Remove the steak to a platter and allow to rest for 5 minutes before cutting. When cutting, using a sharp knife and slice against the grain.

SMOKE

Preheat your smoker for a 230 degrees F cook, and put the steak(s) on the grates. If your smoker has a water pan, make sure that it's full so the smoker doesn't get dry.

Smoke meat 1 hour for every 1.5 pounds of meat, or until steak reaches 125* F using a probe thermometer.

AIR FRY

Air fryers recently became popular and on carnivore we love them! An air fryer is a small convection oven- it cooks at a high temperature with a fan, so the whole steak cooks quickly and evenly.

Cleanup tips: Line the bottom bowl (not the basket) with aluminum foil for easy cleanup. Put a couple tablespoons of water on top of the foil, this will prevent the air fryer from smoking too much.

To air-fry steaks: Preheat air fryer at 400 degrees for 5 minutes. Add 1-2 tablespoons water to the bottom of the fryer to prevent smoking. Salt steak and place in air-fryer basket. Cook at 400* F for 7 minutes on each side, then remove and let rest another 5 minutes before cutting.

INSTANT POT

Where the Air Fryer uses dry heat and air circulation, the Instant Pot uses the power of steam and pressure to quickly and easily cook steaks. This makes 'grey steak' that is the least attractive, but it's delicious. The Instant Pot easily turns gristle and connective tissue into buttery collagen-rich goodness.

To Instant Pot Steaks: Place steak (s) at the bottom of your Instant Pot. Sprinkle with salt. Add 1 cup of water and cook for 45 minutes to obliterate all gristle and turn it into delicious nourishment.

SOUS VIDE

Sous Vide: Ever wonder how high-end restaurant steaks are perfectly pink throughout, with a nice charred crust? The trick is the sous vide! Sous vide is a machine that keeps water at a consistent temperature. Like a little mini hottub for your kitchen.

To Sous Vide Steaks: Set at 130* F vacuum-packaged or plastic-wrapped steak can be cooked medium-rare in the water for 2 hours or all day (like a slow cooker), without over cooking since they never get above 130 degrees, or whatever your desired temperature is.

After removing the fully-cooked steak from the package, you then can sear it quickly (45 seconds a side) in a very hot skillet and serve in minutes.

Sous Vide cookers are about the size of an immersion blender and use a pot filled with water in your kitchen to cook.

NOT COOKED AT ALL

Raw Meat: Taboo, and not for the faint of heart, but many carnivores switch over to occasionally, or primarily, consuming raw beef. When stomach acid is at a low enough PH (low ph = more acidity) humans are well suited to digest beef and other meat raw.

Raw steak, chopped up and lightly salted is the most whole fast food on the carnivore diet. In the wild, carnivores (like dogs and cats) consume all their meat raw, and without chewing. Some human carnivores also choose to include raw meat in their diet.

I too have switched to more raw meat when the weather warms up. I usually cut it into small cubes and chew it just enough to get it down. I was apprehensive the first time I tried raw beef, but I'm confident in my beef source (organic grassfed on lots of pasture, see the resource page for where I get my beef) and it's steadily become a staple in my diet. What does it taste like? It's like the first time you taste sushi - not nearly as strong of a flavor as you'd expect! Raw beef tastes almost buttery, and when it's cold the flavor is even more mild than when it's cooked.

*This cannot be taken as advice, and you need to decide what is healthy for yourself, depending on your own comfort level, quality of meat, and your own immune system/stomach acid level. *

Grilled Salmon

Salmon is a lighter meat, perfect for breakfast!

6-ounce salmon fillet, with skin

sea salt to taste

Grill method: Preheat grill to medium high heat - 400* F or where you can only hold your hand 3" above the grill for 2-4 seconds. As you wait for the grill to preheat (approx 5-10 mins, depending on outside temp) salt the meat on both sides.

Place salmon on the grill skin-side down and grill for 4-5 minutes, then flip with a large thin spatula and cook it for 1 more minute. Salmon is done when it starts to feel firm. It can be under-done and will continue cooking as it cools.

Cast Iron Pan Method: Preheat cast iron pan to medium high heat - if you're not sure, go higher. Preheat for at least 5 minutes. Pat salmon dry and sprinkle with sea salt.

Cook, skin side down for 5-6 minutes, then flip with a large thin spatula and cook it for 1 more minute. Salmon is done when it starts to feel firm. It can be under-done and will continue cooking as it cools.

Poached, Not Grilled: Bring a quart of water or salted stock to a simmer in a saucepan that will fit the salmon fillet in it.

Lower thawed fish in and sprinkle with 1/2 teaspoon sea salt. Turn off heat as soon as the fish is in, and cover. Allow to cook in the hot water, covered, for 20-30 minutes. Drain and serve, sprinkling with additional salt if desired.

Nutrition: 8 oz salmon fillet, with skin:
280 calories, 15 g fat, 0 g carb, 36 g protein

Brisket and Tallow

Brisket is even better leftover than it was the first day! Once shredded, it's like little noodles of delicious meat. See directions here for options to reheat for maximum yum to minimum effort.

8 ounces brisket, leftover from Sunday

1 tablespoon tallow

sea salt

Reheating options for brisket:

Add beef stock to make a soup: stirring brisket into hot stock and then adding salt and tallow .

Pan fry: Melt tallow in a skillet over medium heat. Spread shredded brisket evenly over hot tallow and allow to cook 5 minutes, or until crunchy and starting to brown on the bottom and warm but still tender on the top. Serve, scraping browned bits from the skillet, onto a plate and sprinkle with salt.

Nutrition for 8 ounces brisket + 1 tablespoon tallow:
576 calories, 64 fat, 0 carb, 40 g protein

SEASONING SUGGESTIONS:

Garlic can be added to everything today with delicious results!

Poached Salmon: Simmer 1 bay leaf and 5 peppercorns with the fish. Add a squeeze of lemon when serving.

Adding fresh snipped basil and thyme to the meatballs in addition to garlic adds more flavor with little extra work.

Meatballs and Tallow

Meatballs are perfect traveling food, or for an easy dinner. Meatballs are also great for using game meat (elk, venison) or other combinations of meat - chicken, pork, even salmon!

1-1/2 pounds (12 ounces) ground beef (half for tomorrow)
1 tablespoon tallow
Sea salt to taste

Mix sea salt into ground beef. Roll meat firmly into desired-size meatballs.

Stove top: Heat tallow in a large skillet over medium heat. Add in meatballs so they form a single layer with some space between and use a spatula to turn every 3-4 minutes until all edges are browned and meatballs are cooked, about 12 minutes total. Serve, sprinkling with more salt if desired.

Broiler (oven): Preheat broiler to medium-high. Melt tallow on a broiler-proof shallow-sided baking tray. Line baking tray with meatballs, it's okay if the sides are touching. Broil 4 minutes until outsides start to brown, and inside is no longer pink, turning if needed and broiling for another 4 minutes.

Freezer Cooking Suggestions:

If making extra meatballs to freeze, under cook so the meatballs are still pink in the middle and then cool on a plate. Transfer to zip-top bags or desired freezer container.

To reheat, thaw overnight and then melt some fat in a skillet and add meatballs, saute for 5 minutes or until heated through. Re-heating goes faster with lid.

Nutrition for 3/4 pound ground beef and tallow: 737 calories, 50 g fat, 70 g protein.

Day Total:
1773 calories, 1 g carb, 129 g fat, 145 g protein.

34% calories from protein 66% calories from fat

Lamb Chops

Lamb is often easier to find grassfed/grass finished than beef. Lamb is a nutrient-dense change from beef that is so delicious and easy to prepare!

1 teaspoon fat (tallow, etc)
8 ounce lamb chop
Sea Salt to taste

Grill method: Preheat grill to medium high heat - 400* F or where you can only hold your hand 3" above the grill for 2-4 seconds. As you wait for the grill to preheat (approx 5-10 mins, depending on outside temp) salt the meat on both sides.

Place lamb chop on the grill, and grill for 3-4 minutes. Flip, and grill for an additional 2-3 minutes.

If using a thermometer, grill to 110 for rare, or 130 for medium rare. Meat will continue to raise in temperature as it rests.

Remove the lamb chop(s) to a platter and allow to rest for 5 minutes before cutting. When cutting, using a sharp knife and slice against the grain. Top with tallow for extra fats.

Broiler Method: Preheat broiler to high. Line a broiler-proof baking sheet (most metal baking sheets will be fine, ceramic or glass usually is not) with shallow sides with aluminum foil for easy cleanup.

Salt lamb chop and place on the baking sheet. Broil for 5 minutes on each side, or until internal temperature reaches 110-130*F for rare-med. Allow to rest for 5 minutes before serving.   Top with tallow for extra fats.

Nutrition: 8 oz lamb and 1 teaspoon tallow:
598 calories, 48 g fat, 0 g carb, 38 g protein

Beef Brisket

Reheat 8 ounces brisket and add tallow to taste.

Reheat in the microwave, or by pan-frying in tallow as desired.

Nutrition for 8 ounces brisket + 1 teaspoon tallow:
740 calories, 0 g carb, 63 fat,, 40 g protein

Meatballs and Stock

Simmer your meatballs from yesterday in stock for

Leftover meatballs (3/4 pound)
1-1/2 cups broth

Heat up meatballs by simmering in stock and eat as a soup.

Nutrition for 8 ounces ground beef and 1-1/2 cups beef broth: 620 calories, 0 carb, 47 g fat, 53 g protein

EGG SHELL CALCIUM:

Meat does contain calcium, and it is thought to be an optimized form for human absorption. Still, some people are concerned about lack of calcium when avoiding dairy products on the carnivore diet. Another very well absorbed and nearly free way to supplement calcium is to use egg shells! Really!

To make egg shell calcium: Wash eggs well before cracking if they are unwashed. Save egg shells. Bake shells parchment paper at 350* for 15 minutes, and then crush with a mortar and pestle. 1 teaspoon of powdered egg shell contains approx 1,000 mg calcium. Supplement as needed.
As with most supplements, your individual needs will vary.

Most people can get all the calcium they need from meat only!

Bonus Recipe:
Ground Beef Jerky

This recipe is not reflected in the nutrition facts on this menu, so if you make it and are tracking nutrients, be sure to add the nutrition facts into your daily intake. This recipe uses a dehydrator, I like making jerky in the Excalibur Dehydrator because the square removable trays can hold lots at once. See Resource Page for recommended dehydrator.

2 pounds ground beef
2 tablespoons sea salt

In a bowl, with your hands mix salt into the beef until evenly distributed. Divide beef mixture into 3 or 4 sections. Roll to the size of your dehydrator trays between either paraflex sheets or plastic wrap if you don't have paraflex sheets.
Remove plastic wrap as you flip the meat onto the dehydrator trays.

Score into jerky-sized strips with a sharp knife, being careful not to cut the dehydrator tray, and dry on high overnight, or until thoroughly cooked. Break apart at the score lines. Jerky will be crunchy at this point, and can be spread with soft tallow for a high-fat carnivore boost of energy, or enjoyed on its own for a protein-rich chip alternative.

Store in the fridge or freezer in an air-tight container for up to 12 months. **Makes 20 servings.**

* This Jerky recipe has a complementary video on YouTube

Nutrition per 1 serving jerky:
115 calories, 0 g carb, 9 fat, 7 g protein

Bonus Recipe:
Baked Ghee

Ghee is made from butter, but has all the proteins and lactose removed, making it unlikely to cause problems in those who react to dairy. For nutrition, it is recommended to use butter made from cows raised on pasture. The butter will be a rich golden color, and so will the ghee!

1 pound butter

Preheat oven to 140-250°. Place butter in an ovenproof dish or pan.

Bake for 45-60 minutes, take out very carefully, and pour the golden fat from the top, being careful to leave the white milk solids in the pan.

Keep in a glass jar and use in place of butter.

You can save the buttery milk solids for others who eat butter in the house, or discard.

* This ghee recipe has a complementary video on YouTube

Prepare:

Soak Liver: *Drain any blood from one ounce thawed liver. (you may wish to soak 1 whole pound for use later) Place in a bowl. Cover with filtered water until the liver is completely covered. Cover bowl with lid or plastic wrap and return to the refrigerator.*

Day Total:
1561 calories, 4 g carb, 108 g fat, 139 g protein
1% carb, 63% fat, 36% protein

Sliced Beef Heart

Beef heart is high in CoQ10, the anti-aging vitamin! CoQ10 is associated with cardiovascular health and reducing inflammation. It also is very mild tasting, inexpensive, and easy to prepare!

1 beef heart (approx 3-4 lbs) or 8 ounces as called for in this meal plan this week.
1 teaspoon sea salt
2 cups filtered water

Instant Pot
If not cut in half, cut beef heart in half and remove any hard bits (it may already be trimmed and there is nothing to do). Place in the Instant Pot and sprinkle with sea salt. Pour water around the salted beef heart.

Place the lid on the Instant Pot, and set to 'seal'. Cook on high pressure for 75 minutes on high pressure. Allow pressure to release naturally for at least 15 minutes.

Slow Cooker
Follow the above directions as per the Instant Pot, but cook on low for 8-10 hours in the slow cooker instead of using the pressure setting.

To serve, either method: Slice thinly against the grain, salt as desired, and enjoy warm or cool.

> Nutrition: 4 ounces beef heart: 130 calories, 0 g carb, 5 g fat, 20 g protein

Pork Cracklins, Beef Stock, and Ground Beef Soup

This simple food combination is silky-smooth and salty (stock), meaty and satisfying (beef) and crunchy (cracklins). It's also super easy to prepare ahead of time and pack in a thermos.

1 ounce pork cracklins or pork rinds
2 cups homemade beef stock
1/2 pound ground beef
Sea salt to taste

Simmer beef patties in stock and then pack into thermoses if desired, or eat as soup. Alternatively, eat the meat patties and drink the stock. Cracklins can be used as croûtons in the soup or eaten on their own.

> Nutrition for 1 ounce pork cracklins, 2 cups beef stock and 8 ounces ground beef: 757 calories, 0 g carb, 48 g fat, 81 g protein

SEASONING SUGGESTIONS:

Slices of heart can be dipped in mustard, especially spicy flavored mustard!

Ginger and chives are delicious added to lunch's beef stock.

Garlic is a great cover up flavor for liver, so if you are eating seasonings and want to eat more liver, add 2-3 garlic cloves to the liver and beef meatballs or patties.

Superfood Beef Liver Meatballs or Patties

Liver is such a good source of A, B, and D vitamins, iron, and more that it should be consumed regularly on the carnivore diet. Here we introduce a little liver into our ground beef to cut the strong flavor.

Even if you didn't soak your liver last night, you can still rinse it off under cool running water and get this recipe on the table for dinner tonight!

1/2 pound ground beef
1 ounce beef liver
1 tablespoon tallow
Sea salt to taste

Finely chop liver and mix into ground beef along with sea salt. Form into patties or meatballs Fry patties in tallow over medium heat, leaving slightly undercooked.

Enjoy this superfood and the energy it gives you!

Nutrition for Superfood Beef Liver Meatballs or Patties above:
573 calories, 1 g carb, 38 g fat, 55 g protein

Day Total:
1804 calories, 1 g carb, 104 g fat, 209 g protein
57% fat 43% protein

Sautéed Shrimp

Change up the flavor and texture with a side of shrimp. Surf and turf is the classic pairing of red meat and seafood. Here we serve them alongside Superfood Patties, but they are a perfect side dish for any meat.

1/2 pound wild-caught shrimp, deveind, tails removed.
1 tablespoon tallow (or ghee)
sea salt to taste

Heat a skillet over medium heat, and melt tallow. Add shrimp, frozen or thawed. If cooking from frozen, the process will be faster if you cook for the first 5 minutes with a lid over your skillet.

From thawed, shrimp only take minutes to cook - cook until they start to turn bright pink, and become firm. They will continue cooking slightly once removed from heat. Cooking time depends on how large the shrimp are.

Nutrition for Shrimp: 334 calories, 0 g carb, 13 g fat, 53 g protein

Start for tomorrow: Prepare roast and/or ribs for the Instant Pot or slow cooker.

Please note, if you have leftover brisket you can continue eating that.

If you have to cook both ribs and a roast, you can do both in the Instant Pot or slow cooker at the same time.

Pork Sausage

When selecting pork sausage at the store, look for plain ground pork (and possibly salt) as the only ingredient. Often preservatives or fillers sneak into ground pork.

If you're ordering pork from heritage pigs (as with Butcher Box or US Wellness Meats) the meat may appear darker than you're used to. This is due to a different breed of pork, and the meat is so much more flavorful and nutrient-dense.

1 pound ground pork
Sea Salt to taste

Form ground pork into patties and sprinkle with sea salt.

Heat a skillet or griddle over medium heat and grease with bacon fat or other cooking fat. Once hot, form meat mixture into patties and fry until no longer pink in the center if eating immediately, or still slightly pink if storing to reheat later.

For crumbled sausage, brown, breaking up chunks with a spatula as you cook it.

Reserve half pork sausage for tomorrow.

> Nutrition: 8 oz pork sausage:
> 594 calories, 0 g carb, 48 g fat, 38 g protein

> **Prepare extra for easy meals:** Looking for good food on the run? Superfood Beef Liver patties are easy to pre-cook and are good cold! I'm partial to doing a whole mess of them on the grill and then grabbing as needed from the fridge, but they can certainly be cooked in batches on the stovetop instead.

Beef Roast & Stock

You probably still have brisket leftover, but if other members of your household have demolished it (it's delicious! Who could blame them?!) then we'll go ahead and make a chuck roast today. Ribs and Roast can be done in the slow cooker at the same time if your slow cooker is large enough. See tomorrow's page for a pork butt roast if you're looking for something other than more beef.

1 cup beef stock
3 pound beef chuck roast
Sea Salt to taste

Instant Pot:
Sprinkle roast with sea salt on all sides. Pour filtered water in the pot of the Instant Pot.
Cook at high pressure (manual) for 90 minutes and allow pressure to release naturally for at least 20 minutes, then use quick release to release the rest of the pressure.

Slow Cooker:
Prepare as for the Instant Pot, but cook on low for 6-8 hours. Roast is done when the meat around the edges is starting to be able to be shredded, but the whole roast doesn't fall apart when you pick it up with tongs.

Continue for either way of cooking:
Allow to rest for 10 minutes on the cutting board before slicing. Allow cooking liquid to set, and skim fat to use in cooking or add all the liquid to your beef stock
Cut across the grain into thin slices and top with stock that includes fat from cooking, and salt.

> Nutrition for 8 ounces chuck roast with 2 cups beef stock:
> 720 calories, 0 g carb, 50 g fat, 62 g protein

Beef or Pork Ribs

Ribs make more stock as they cook. I like them best cooked completely under liquid as described in this recipe, but your preferences may vary. Low and slow cooking is the key to turning ribs into the melt-in-your mouth treat that you will love!

2 pounds beef or pork ribs, bone-in (reserve half for tomorrow's lunch)
1 cup beef stock (optional)
1 tablespoon sea salt
Water to cover

Place ribs in the slow cooker or Instant Pot, along with beef stock (optional), sea salt, and water. Cook on low all day, the longer the better! In the Instant pot, cook on high pressure for 90 minutes.

Strain out stock from cooking and add salt to taste. Keep stock in the fridge.

Makes approx 1 pound of meat; **2 servings,** for today and tomorrow

Nutrition for 1/2 lb (8 oz- meat only, no bones) beef ribs 340 calories, 0 g carb, 26 g fat, 36 g protein

SEASONING SUGGESTIONS:

To the sausage, add 1/4 teaspoon each: coriander, dried sage, fennel, and dried parsley, and a small pinch of cayenne pepper.

To ribs, barbecue sauce of choice can be added before slow cooking, in place of the water to cover.

WHY SO MUCH RED MEAT?

Most people find that they feel best when eating red meat on carnivore vs poultry or fish. The reason for this is because cows in particular have such a long digestive system, allowing them to extract even more nutrition out of plants as they turn them into meat. Second, chickens are commonly supplemented with corn and soy, common allergens that may affect some 'second hand'.

Day Total:
1654 calories, 0 g carb, 38 g fat, 42 g protein 67% fat 33% fat

Pork Sausage and Beef Stock

If you're abstaining from coffee, salted beef stock replaces the warm morning ritual while providing essential electrolytes, amino acids, and fats to start the day. Pork sausage is a familiar breakfast food to fill your stomach for the day.

4 ounces pork sausage (leftover from yesterday)
2 cups homemade beef stock

Reheat Sausage
Grease a pan lightly fat tallow or other fat, and then fry pork sausage over medium-low heat until

Heat stock in microwave or in a saucepan over medium heat, adding salt to taste.

Nutrition for sausage and stock:
497 calories, 36 fat, 0 carb, 39 g protein

Leftover Ribs

1/2 pound ribs, leftover
Sea Salt

Reheat ribs in the microwave or with a little water in a saucepan, covered, over medium heat.

Nutrition for 1/2 lb (8 oz) beef ribs 340 calories, 0 g carb, 26 g fat, 36 g protein

Beef Roast

Reheat roast by pan-frying in tallow, simmering in drippings, or heating in the microwave.

8 ounces beef roast
2 cups stock/drippings

Nutrition for 8 ounces chuck roast with 2 cups beef stock:
685 calories, 0 g carb, 34 g fat, 47 g protein

SEASONING SUGGESTIONS:

Garlic, ginger, and cayenne are flavorful additions to beef stock.

Drippings from roast make an amazing gravy, thickened with pureed cooked onions if grain-free or with a traditional roux.

Garlic, onion, apple cider vinegar, and BBQ sauce all can be added to roast before or after cooking/shredding.

Day Total:
1715 calories, 0 g carb, 115 g fat, 155 g protein
63% calories from fat 37 % calories from protein

BEYOND TABLE SALT

Sea salt is recommended on the carnivore diet for trace minerals. Other useful salts on the carnivore diet are Epsom salt (for soaking) and potassium chloride.

Table salt almost always has iodine added to it. When we purchase 'dirty' sea salt, which is dehydrated sea water, we get natural iodine and other trace minerals from the sea. When choosing salt, choose Redmond's Sea Salt, Celtic Sea Salt, or Himalayan Pink Salt.

In addition, essential electrolytes (other salts) that you may need to supplement as you adjust to the carnivore diet are magnesium and potassium.

For potassium, potassium chloride tastes like table salt and can be found as a salt substitute 'No Salt' at most major grocery stores.

Magnesium can be upsetting to the digestive tract, so an easy way to get magnesium without harming your guts is to plug up the tub while you shower and add 1/2 cup of Epsom salt to the bottom of the tub. Your feet will absorb what you need. Magnesium and sulfur (both in Epsom salt - magnesium sulfate) are both commonly low in the modern population. Previously, we got lots of minerals from untreated water and walking with the dirt (which also contains minerals!) right against our skin.

Other ways to absorb minerals are to soak in natural hotsprings. If you live in an area with natural hotsprings, soaking allows your skin to absorb needed minerals, and mimics the time when we were bathing and washing in mineral water with every day.

BEYOND TAP OR BOTTLED WATER

Filtered water is recommended on the carnivore diet unless you are on a well with untreated water that is safe to drink. I recommend the Berkey water filter, see the resource page for links. Tap water contains chlorine, which adds toxins, increasing your toxic load. Many bottled waters aren't any different than tap water.

In addition to chlorine, in many areas tap water contains trace pharmaceuticals that have not been adequately been filtered out at the water treatment plant. Fluoride is also added to many public water sources.

Here is an excerpt from a medical journal discussion (source below) on fluoride:

"Fluoride has modest benefit in terms of reduction of dental caries but significant costs in relation to cognitive impairment, hypothyroidism, dental and skeletal fluorosis, enzyme and electrolyte derangement, and uterine cancer. Given that most of the toxic effects of fluoride are due to ingestion, whereas its predominant beneficial effect is obtained via topical application, ingestion or inhalation of fluoride predominantly in any form constitutes an unacceptable risk with virtually no proven benefit."

If not fluoride, how do you protect your teeth? By eating nutrient-dense foods (like meat and dairy!) that provide the body with needed nutrients to form healthy teeth and repair dental caries (cavities).

Last, you may have been told to drink water until your urine is clear. For many people, that is too much hydration. It is recommend to drink to thirst, and keep water drinking during meals to a minimum so as to not dilute stomach acid.

Sources:

https://www.ncbi.nlm.nih.gov/pubmed/18782969
price-pottenger.org
https://www.ncbi.nlm.nih.gov/pmc/articles/PMC3956646/
https://www.ncbi.nlm.nih.gov/pubmed/18473176

CARNIVORE   MEAT & EGGS

SUNDAY
- **B**   STEAK, BACON, AND FRIED EGG
- **L**   CARNIVORE SANDWICH
- **D**   PORK BUTT ROAST

MONDAY
- **B**   EGGS FRIED IN TALLOW
- **L**   SASHIMI WITH EGG YOLK
- **D**   HAMBURGERS WITH BACON

TUESDAY
- **B**   SCOTCH EGGS
- **L**   LEFTOVER BURGER PATTIES AND BACON
- **D**   TRITIP

WEDNESDAY
- **B**   TRITIP, WITH EGG
- **L**   LIVER PATE AND PORK RINDS OR CRACKLINS
- **D**   LEFTOVER TRITIP, SAUTEED IN TALLOW

THURSDAY
- **B**   SCOTCH EGG
- **L**   TRITIP, LIVER PATE, AND EGG
- **D**   INSTANT POT HEART

FRIDAY
- **B**   LEFTOVER HEART AND EGGS WITH BACON SPRINKLES
- **L**   EGG SALAD WITH BACONAISE
- **D**   NY STRIP STEAK WITH FRIED EGG

SATURDAY
- **B**   BACON
- **L**   NY STRIP STEAK WITH EGGS
- **D**   ROTISSERIE CHICKEN & BROTH

MEAL PLAN

GROCERY *List*

- ☐ Pork, ground, 2 lbs
- ☐ Pork, butt roast, 3 lbs
- ☐ Bacon 1-2 lbs
- ☐ Sashimi, 6 oz
- ☐ Anchovies, jarred, 2 oz
- ☐ Beef, flat iron steak, 6 oz
- ☐ Beef, ground, 1-1/2 lbs
- ☐ Beef, heart, 8 oz
- ☐ Beef, tritip, 2.5-3 lbs
- ☐ Beef, NY Strip 16 oz (2 total)
- ☐ Chicken, rotisserie, 1
- ☐ Chicken, liver, 1 lb
- ☐ Sea Salt, 1 cup
- ☐ Eggs, 4 dozen
- ☐ Pork Rinds, 2 oz

Carnivore Breakfast Sandwich

Meat is your new bread! And with an egg between (runny yolk, please) you're in breakfast sandwich heaven!

4 ounces ground pork
1 egg
1 tablespoon bacon grease or beef tallow

Form ground pork into 2 large flat patties and sprinkle with sea salt.

Heat a skillet or griddle over medium heat and grease with fat. Once hot, form meat mixture into patties and fry until no longer pink in the center. Set sausage patties aside.

Add more fat if needed, and fry one egg so that the white is set and the yolk is still runny. Sandwich fried egg between two cooked sausage patties and enjoy.

Using a well-seasoned cast iron pan will produce the best sausage and eggs. However, stainless can be washed in the dishwasher and is lighter to move around the kitchen. To keep eggs from sticking in either case, grease and preheat pan well. The do not attempt to flip egg until there are bubbles under the entire egg white.

Nutrition: per breakfast sandwich
503 calories, 0 g carb, 44 g fat, 25 g protein

Steak, Bacon, and Fried Egg

3 pieces bacon
Flat iron steak, 6 ounces

1 egg

Cook bacon in a cast iron skillet over medium heat, remove while still slightly soft. Raise heat to medium high and sear steak. Once the first side is seared, flip, and lower heat to medium-low. Continue cooking for 5 minutes, or to desired doneness. Fry egg as the steak rests, and re-heat bacon as the egg fries in the same pan. .

If you're going to try doing a steak in the Instant Pot (directions on page 31), this is a great one to start with. Instant Potting this steak ensures the connective tissue is soft and easy to eat. Covering with a glistening fried egg and crisp bacon can help the less-than-beautiful presentation of an Instant Pot steak.

Nutrition for steak, bacon, and egg as above: 444 calories, 2 g carb, 25 g fat, 25 g protein

Shredded Pork Butt Roast

Pork butt roast is a great roast to make once and then enjoy for days! The meat shreds beautifully, and freezes well as well.

Pork butt roast, approx 3 pounds
1 cup stock or water
1 tablespoon sea salt
1 tablespoon tallow

Instant Pot: In Instant Pot, turn to saute-medium and melt tallow. Once preheated, brown pork roast on all sides, about 5-10 minutes each. Sprinkle with sea salt and then add stock or water to the Instant Pot. Cook on high pressure (manual) for 1 hour 15 minutes and then allow pressure to release naturally (this will take another 45ish minutes).

Slow cooker: Brown pork roast on the stove top in a large cast iron skillet and then transfer to slow cooker and sprinkle with salt. Omit stock/water. Cook on low for 8-10 hours.

Either method: Once roast has cooked, it should fall apart when pressure is applied. If it doesn't, return to cook longer. Allow to cool until comfortable to touch. Using two forks, or using a hand-held or stand mixer (Yes! this works), shred meat.

To eat: Pour juices (stir the fats back in) over shredded meat and add salt to taste.

Another method (my favorite!) is to pan-fry shredded pork in hot oil. Preheat fat in a skillet over medium-high heat, making sure it's well preheated. Drop pieces of shredded meat in the hot oil until the bottom of the pan is covered in meat, like a meat pancake. Cook on one side until the bottom starts to get crisp, and the top part is heated through. Then use a thin metal spatula to fold in half, like an omelet, and serve. Meat should be tender and soft inside, and crispy on the outside - yum!

Nutrition for 8 ounces pork butt roast with 1/2 cup juices/stock and 1 tablespoon fat: 773 calories, 0 g carb, 59 g fat, 58 g protein

SEASONING SUGGESTIONS:

To the pork sausage for breakfast, add 1/4 teaspoon each: coriander, dried sage, fennel, and dried parsley, and a small pinch of cayenne pepper.

To roast, a jar of tomato sauce tenderizes and adds flavor. Pour over before cooking (either method). Crushed garlic (3 cloves) and freshly ground black pepper also are delicious. Use those along with or instead of the tomato sauce.

Day Total:
1670 calories, 2 g carb, 125 g fat, 103 g protein

73% calories from fat
27% calories from protein

Eggs Fried in Tallow

3 eggs
1 tablespoon tallow or other fat
Sea salt to taste

In a skillet over medium-high heat, melt tallow or other fat. Crack eggs into fat and flip once the underside of the eggs start to bubble. Cook briefly on the other side, just long enough to cook the egg white.

> Nutrition for 3 eggs fried in tallow:
> 388 calories, 31 g fat, 1 g carb, 25 g protein

EGGS ALWAYS STICKING TO YOUR STAINLESS STEEL SKILLET?

Cleanup tip after cooking eggs: If you cook eggs in a stainless steel skillet and notice that it's hard to clean, before you serve the eggs, run your kitchen faucet on hot to get hot water. Immediately after removing eggs to a plate, drop a drop of dish soap into the hot pan, and then fill to cover the stuck egg-bits with hot water. Return to the (still warm, but off) burner as you eat. After sitting, any stuck egg will release immediately!

Have a stainless steel pan that has burnt-on food stains? Another trick is to fill with hot water, and then add 1/4 cup salt evenly over the pan. Simmer for 10 minutes, allow to cool, and the stains will wipe right off with a kitchen sponge!

Sashimi and Raw Egg Yolks

Not ready for raw egg yolks and raw fish? Heat up some of your shredded pork from yesterday instead or poach salmon and 2 whole eggs.

4 egg yolks
6 ounces Sashimi (sushi-grade tuna or other fish)

Cut sashimi into bite-sized pieces and salt to taste. Add egg yolks and stir to create a sauce.

Raw is easy and doesn't require reheating. As long as you can keep your yolks and fish chilled, like with an ice pack, this is a great packed lunch!

> Nutrition for sashimi and egg yolks:
> 465 calories, 2 g carb, 27 g fat, 51 g protein

FLAVOR ADDITIONS:

Fried Eggs: A squeeze of lemon is a surprising and delicious finish to fried eggs! You may never want to go back.

Sashimi: Coconut aminos provide salty umami flavor without soy.

Burgers: Sprinkle with chili powder for a kick.

Burgers with Bacon

Here we go! If you need more calories, add a fried egg to this too.

3 pieces bacon

1-1/2 pounds ground beef (reserve half for tomorrow)

In a skillet over medium heat, fry bacon. Remove the bacon once slightly under-done (it will continue cooking as it cools), leaving grease in the pan. Use the bacon grease to fry the burgers.

To fry burgers, heat skillet up to medium-high and then sear burgers on the first side. Flip, and lower heat to medium-low to cook the other side and continue cooking through to desired doneness.

Top burgers with cooked bacon, or chop up bacon for 'bacon sprinkles'.

Nutrition for 3 pieces bacon and 3/4 lbs ground beef: 727 calories, 2 g carb, 47 g fat, 78 g protein

Day Total:
1580 calories, 5 g carb, 108 g fat, 147 g protein

1% calories from carb, 62% calories from fat 37% calories from protein

PREPARE:

Soft boiled eggs for Scotch Eggs (see recipe tomorrow) are super fast food when you prepare them ahead of time.

At the least, you'll want to soft-cook the eggs tonight in preparation for tomorrow.

Instant Pot: Cook eggs on a trivet or in a steamer basket in the Instant Pot for 3 minutes on high pressure, then quick release and plunge into a large bowl of ice cold water to cool immediately.

Stove Top: Cook eggs on the stove top by placing in a saucepan covered with cold water to the top. Bring to a boil over high heat, and once the water comes to a boil, boil for 3 minutes. Immediately plunge cooked eggs into a large bowl of ice cold water after the 2 minutes.

INSTANT POT TIP:

The silicone seal in the Instant Pot lid need to be replaced approximately every 25 uses. If your eggs aren't cooking enough in 2-3 minutes, it's likely because your seal needs to be replaced.

Scotch Eggs

These scotch eggs are so fun to make, and are a perfectly portable and filling take-along meal. Traditionally a picnic food from London, the scotch egg is served with mustard, these are also delicious with a mixture of horseradish and yogurt, or on their own.

4 eggs
1 pound pork sausage (ground pork)
2 cups pork rinds

Cook your eggs to desired doneness. (Directions on previous day)

Peel cooked eggs and chill, uncovered, for at least an hour in the refrigerator. This helps the exterior to dry out so the sausage will stick without needing a starch to bind.
As the eggs chill, crush pork rinds by placing in a heavy duty zip-top bag and crushing well with a rolling pin or pulse in a food processor until fine crumbs are made.

After the eggs have chilled, divide pork sausage into 8 even pieces. To cover each egg, carefully flatten one piece of the divided pork sausage into a round about the size of your palm. Do the same with a second piece of pork sausage.

Place one sausage round in the palm of your hand, then place the egg in the middle. Place the second round on top, and gently press the two rounds together until well covering every part of the egg, making sure to firmly but gently press together all seams.

Repeat with the remaining eggs and sausage.
Place crushed pork rinds in a soup bowl or shallow dish and roll sausage-covered eggs in the pork rinds. Again, with your hands, firmly but carefully press pork rinds into the sausage mixture, so it evenly coats the egg.

Cook in Airfryer: Preheat the airfryer to 375* F. Line the bottom under the basket with foil if desired to make cleanup easier. Once the airfryer has preheated, place 2-3 eggs in the basket and air fry for 15 minutes. When done, the outside of the scotch egg will be starting to darken and the pork sausage will no longer be pink next to the hard-cooked egg. Repeat with the remaining eggs.

Cook in Oven: Preheat oven to 400* F. Place Scotch Eggs on a baking sheet and bake for 25 minutes, turning once to prevent the bottoms from getting soggy.

Serve immediately or keep at room temperature for 2-3 hours before serving (as in packing for lunch).

* This recipe has a complementary video on YouTube

Nutrition in each Scotch Egg:
542 calories, 45 g fat, 2 g carb, 31 g protein

Leftover Burger Patties and Bacon

2 pieces bacon
3/4 pound ground beef (you should have leftovers from yesterday)

Quick and easy, reheating in a pan or air fryer helps keep this meal crispy, but a microwave works in a pinch.

Nutrition:
687 calories, 1 g carb, 43 g fat, 75 g protein

Tritip

Tritip roast is one of the more flavorful less-expensive cuts of meat. Mastering your tritip game is a skill you want to develop- this cut of meat is not only perfect for the carnivore diet, but it is great for feeding company as well.

2.5-3-pound tritip (8 ounces for today)
1 tablespoon tallow (oven recipe)
sea salt to taste

Grilled Tritip: For best results, allow beef to come to room temperature before cooking (sit out for 1 hour). Salt meat liberally on all sides.
Preheat the grill to medium-high. Grill for 5 minutes per side over medium-high heat to make a beautiful crust, flipping only once. Remove to indirect heat (move the roast so that it isn't over the coals or the lit burner) and continue cooking until internal temperature is 130* F for medium rare, about 10-15 more minutes.

Oven Tritip: Preheat your oven to 425°F. and sprinkle meat on all sides with sea salt. Heat a large oven-safe skillet over high heat until very hot. Add tallow and then as soon as the tallow melts, sear meat on both sides. Leave fat-side up and roast in oven for **10 minutes per pound** until internal temperature reaches 130* F.

Either Method: Remove meat to rest on a platter for at least 10 minutes before slicing in thin slices across the grain to serve.

Slow cooker Tritip: Salt tritip and then cook on high for 4-5 hours, or low for 8-10 hours. Reserve juices and fat to pour over meat. Shred with forks, adding juices back in to shredded meat.

PREPARE:

Soak Liver for tomorrow: Drain any blood from 1 pound thawed chicken liver. Place in a bowl.

Cover with filtered water until the liver is completely covered. Cover bowl with lid or plastic wrap and return to the fridge.

Nutrition in 8 ounces tritip:
420 calories, 1 g carb, 31 g fat, 52 g protein

Day Total:
1649 calories 4 g carb, 119 g fat, 158 g protein

2% calories from carb, 64% calories from fat, 34% calories from protein

Tritip and Fried Egg

2 teaspoons beef tallow or other fat
4 ounces tritip
1 egg
Sea salt to taste

Pan-fry leftover chopped tritip in tallow. Remove tritip once warm, leaving tallow in the pan. Use same pan with tallow to fry an egg, and top your leftover tritip. Fast and delicious!

Nutrition:
388 calories, 31 g fat, 1 g carb, 25 g protein

Liver Pate and Pork Rinds or Cracklins

Crunchy and nutrient dense, the perfect combo! 4505 brand makes seasoning-free pork cracklins that are higher in fat, or you can choose Epic Sea Salt Pork Rinds that are more chip-like.

2 ounces Pork Cracklins or Pork Rinds
1 ounce chicken liver pate (see recipe on next page)

Dip pork rinds into chicken liver pate. The liver pate spreads/dips more easily if it is gently heated or sits out for 10 minutes before eating.

Nutrition:
500 calories, 23 fat, 3 carb, 38 g protein

Leftover Tritip and Egg 'Noodle' Soup

We make stock and chopped meat into a little egg-drop soup here. If you want more of a creamy soup base, omit the egg white and use 2-3 yolks instead. Egg yolks in soup make a really nice creamy texture!

2 cups beef stock
Sea salt to taste
1 egg
8 ounces tritip

In a small saucepan, bring stock to a simmer. As the stock heats, chop tritip into small cubes and whisk the egg with a fork in a small bowl.

To make 'egg drop soup' keep the beef stock simmering, and whisk it in a circular motion with a fork or whisk. Slowly drizzle in egg as you continue whisking in the circular motion. Thin 'noodles' should form as the stream of egg cooks in the hot stock.

Add chopped tritip and continue simmering gently until tritip is heated through.

Nutrition:
899 calories, 55 fat, 2 carb, 101 g protein

Chicken Liver Pate

Liver pate is a great way eat liver.   Spread on meat, dip pork rinds in it, and enjoy by the spoonful.

1 pound chicken livers, soaked (see previous day)
Filtered water
1/4 cup tallow
1 two-ounce can of anchovies, drained

Over medium heat in a large saucepan, heat
tallow until melted, then add liver and cook until the
outside is done, but the inside is still pink. Pour all the
melted tallow and cooked liver in a food processor.
To food processor add drained anchovies (if omitting,
add 1 teaspoon sea salt)
Process until well pureed and all of the
ingredients are well combined.
Scoop into ramekins and then top with melted tallow if
desired. Store covered in the freezer for up to 6 months
or in the refrigerator for up to 10 days.

* This recipe has a complementary video on YouTube

Nutrition per ounce:
60 calories, 4 fat, 0 carb, 4 g protein

SEASONING SUGGESTIONS:

Egg 'noodle' soup lends itself well to hot pepper flakes, soy sauce or coconut aminos, and thinly sliced green onions.

To the **Chicken Liver Pate**, make a garlic version by adding in 4 cloves chopped garlic to the tallow and frying til soft, and then adding to the food processor. One teaspoon fresh thyme and 2 tablespoons of cognac or scotch can also be added to the food processor before blending.

WHAT KIND OF LIVER?

Chicken liver is more mild than beef liver, and that's why we choose that variety for the recipe here. When made into pate, it is a delicious introduction to liver. If you didn't grow up eating liver, you may find the taste to be strong.

Keep trying it, and allow your body to respond to the easily absorbable vitamins that are plentiful in liver. You may find that soon you crave (though maybe still don't love) liver!

Scotch Egg

Cook Scotch Egg reserved from Tuesday in the oven or Air Fryer at 400* Or re-heat a cooked Scotch Egg in the microwave for 1:30 on high.

> Nutrition in each Scotch Egg:
> 542 calories, 45 g fat, 2 g carb, 31 g protein

Tritip and Liver Pate

1 teaspoon tallow
8 ounces tritip

1 egg
1 ounce chicken liver pate

In a skillet, melt tallow over medium heat. As the tallow heats, chop tritip. Pan-fry tritip in tallow and then re-move. Fry egg in remaining tallow in the pan, keeping yolk runny. Top tritip with fried egg and then scoop a dollop of pate on top.

Packed lunch version: Eat tritip cold (or microwaved) and have a hard-boiled egg, cut in half and spread with tallow and liver pate.

> Nutrition in lunch: 609 calories, 6 g carb, 40 g fat, 53 g protein

Heart & Eggs

Beef heart is a mild-tasting meat that complements eggs well. Chop it up like you would cube ham, and add to your scrambled eggs.

4 ounces beef heart
3 eggs, scrambled in 1 teaspoon fat
Sea salt to taste

Chop or slice beef heart and top with scrambled eggs. Sprinkle with sea salt to taste.

> Nutrition:
> 403 calories, 26 fat, 2 carb, 38 g protein

> Day Total:
> 1554 calories, 9 g carb, 111 g fat, 122 g protein
>
> 2% calories from carb, 33% calories from protein, 65% calories from fat

Beef Heart Recipe

1 beef heart (approx 3-4 lbs) or 8 ounces as called for in this meal plan this week.
1 teaspoon sea salt
2 cups filtered water

Instant Pot
If not cut in half, cut beef heart in half and remove any hard bits (it may already be trimmed and there is nothing to do). Place in the Instant Pot and sprinkle with sea salt. Pour water around the salted beef heart.

Place the lid on the Instant Pot, and set to 'seal'. Cook on high pressure for 75 minutes on high pressure. Allow pressure to release naturally for at least 15 minutes.

Slice thinly against the grain, salt as desired, and enjoy warm or cool.

Slow Cooker
Follow the above directions as per the Instant Pot, but cook on low for 8-10 hours in the slow cooker instead of using the pressure setting.

Organ meat, also called offal, is a debatable topic among carnivores. Some carnivores insist that nose-to-tail eating is necessary, and care should be taken to add in heart, liver, kidney, even brains, on a regular basis for optimum nutrition. Still others have been doing 'ribeye carnivore' for years, never having felt anything other than fabulous.

Nose-to-tail refers to eating every part of the animal including cartilage, marrow, organs like liver and kidney, and even brains!. While we don't usually literally eat noses, we do eat beef cheeks and oxtail!

Organ meats are fun to experiment with. If you're finding your feel run down, the iron and B vitamins in liver may be just what you need.

If you want anti-aging benefits or improved cardiac health, heart is worth giving a try! Marrow is like the butter of meat, and as far as offal goes, it's probably the easiest to get used to.

EAT IT TO HEAL IT:

If you're eating to heal a certain condition or part of your body, the general rule is to eat the part of the animal that corresponds to that part.

This 'rule' seems too simple to be true, but the science points in this direction too:

- Heart is high in CoQ10, which is important for cardiac function.
- Brain contains choline, specifically phosphatidylcholine which is important for the nervous system.
- Connective tissue around bones is simmered to release essential amino acids to repair our own joints.
- Rocky Mountain Oysters (bull testes) - yes I'm going here - are high in zinc, which supports healthy sex drive and sperm counts in males.
- Placenta consumption has little, if any, formal studies but the vast majority of mothers who consume their placenta following birth report significant benefits.

Sources:
https://www.medicalnewstoday.com/articles/319229.php
https://ods.od.nih.gov/factsheets/Choline-HealthProfessional/#en1
http://www.medsci.org/v06p0312.htm
https://www.ncbi.nlm.nih.gov/pubmed/26268328
https://www.ncbi.nlm.nih.gov/pubmed/30889405
https://www.tandfonline.com/doi/abs/10.1080/03670244.2012.719356

Heart and Eggs with Bacon Sprinkles

2 pieces bacon
3 eggs
4 ounces heart

In a skillet over medium heat, fry bacon. Remove the bacon once slightly under-done (it will continue cooking as it cools), leaving grease in the pan. Use the bacon grease to fry chopped heart, and then add in eggs to make scrambled eggs. Sprinkle with crumbled or chopped bacon.

> Nutrition for Heart and Eggs with Bacon:
> 483 calories, 2 g carb, 33 g fat, 43 g protein

Egg Salad

3 tablespoons bacon mayo (recipe next page)
3 eggs, hard cooked

Make hard-cooked eggs using your method of choice (see column to the right) and peel and chop. Mix with bacon mayo for egg salad, sprinkling with sea salt to taste if needed..

Not making mayonnaise? No problem! Just cut eggs in half, smear with bacon grease, and sprinkle with sea salt. Mmmm...

> Nutrition for egg salad:
> 620 calories, 1 g carb, 60 g fat, 18 g protein

NY Strip Steak with a Fried Egg

Steak and a fried egg is forever satisfying. This is your go-to meal on this week of carnivore, repeat as often as desired!.

1 tablespoon fat
1 egg
8 ounce New York strip steak

Melt grease in a skillet and cook steak. For specifics on the many different ways to cook steak, see page 31. As steak rests, fry egg in leftover drippings and tallow until white is cooked but yolk is still runny. Top steak with egg and enjoy!

> Nutrition for Steak and Eggs:
> 707 calories, 0 g carb, 54 g fat, 52 g protein

> Day Total:
> 1810 calories, 3 g carb, 147 g fat, 113 g protein
>
> 1% calories from carb, 25% calories from protein, 74% calories from fat

Hard-Cooked Eggs

Hard cooking eggs can be done in many ways, they can even be baked! Of all these methods, I find eggs cooked in the Instant Pot to be easiest to peel.

12 eggs

Instant Pot: Cook eggs on a trivet or in a steamer basket in the Instant Pot for 7 minutes on high pressure, then quick release and plunge into a large bowl of ice cold water to cool immediately. Peel once cooled, after about 10 minutes.

Stove Top: Cook eggs on the stove top by placing in a saucepan covered with cold water to the top. Bring to a boil over high heat, and once the water comes to a boil, boil for 10 minutes. Immediately plunge cooked eggs into a large bowl of ice cold water after the 10 minutes.

Baked: Preheat oven to 350* F .
Put 1 egg in each of 12 muffin cups.
Bake in preheated oven for 30 minutes. Plunge baked eggs in a large bowl filled with ice water until cooled completely, about 10 minutes.

Bacon Mayo

Bacon mayonnaise is a high fat creamy condiment made with just egg yolks and bacon grease. If your bacon is particularly salty, omit the salt.

2 egg yolks
¼ teaspoon sea salt
1 cup bacon grease, warmed

Put the egg yolks in the high-powered blender. Blend on medium, until combined.

With blender on high, slowly drizzle in warmed bacon grease, a little bit at a time so that the mixture has time to thicken. Drizzling in should take about 1 minute total.
Continue to blend mixture for another 1-2 minutes, allowing it to thicken.

Transfer to a wide-mouth mason jar, cover and refrigerate. Keep in the fridge up to 5 days.

BACON MAYO FLAVORING OPTIONS:

Add in any or all of the following:
1 tablespoon fresh lemon juice
1 tablespoon white wine vinegar
1 teaspoon Dijon mustard
Black pepper to taste

Bacon

4 pieces bacon

In a skillet over medium heat, fry bacon. Remove the bacon once slightly under-done (it will continue cooking as it cools). Reserve bacon grease for future cooking and bacon mayonnaise.

Nutrition in 4 pieces bacon: 160 calories, 2 g carb, 14 g fat, 10 g protein

NY Strip Steak with 3 Hard Boiled Eggs

Simple and hearty, this lunch will carry you through to dinner. If you don't want hard boiled eggs, go ahead and fry them up in this morning's bacon grease. We don't blame you - we can't get enough steak with a fried egg either.

6 ounce steak, prepared as desired
1 tablespoon bacon grease
3 hard boiled eggs, chopped

Nutrition in steak fried in bacon grease with chopped eggs: 680 calories, 1 g carb, 52 g fat, 52 g protein

Rotisserie Chicken

After a weekend day of play (or chores) an easy dinner is called for. If you don't do your grocery shopping on Saturdays, you may want to swap this meal out and have it on grocery shopping days.

1/2 rotisserie chicken (mostly dark meat)

Enjoy the fatty skin, and mostly dark meat from this chicken. After you've picked the carcass clean, throw it in a stock pot, slow cooker, or Instant Pot (recipe on next page) to extract even more nutrition and enjoy as chicken stock (directions below).

Bare brand rotisserie chickens are available in many grocery stores and don't contain any additives. If you're not completely avoiding all seasonings and spices, the Costco rotisserie chickens can't be beat as far as price goes.

Nutrition: per 3 ounce light meat, 12 ounces dark meat: 700 calories, 0 g carb, 41 g fat, 82 g protein

Day Total:
1539 calories, 3 g protein, 106 g fat, 143 g protein

1% calories from carb, 37% calories from protein, 62% calories from fat

Bonus Recipe: Chicken Broth

Stock is not only highly digestible, but it also is a great way to get extra salt in and something to sip on when cravings strike. These directions are for the Instant Pot, but you can do the same thing in a stock pot - just simmer on low instead of cooking under pressure, or in a slow cooker cook on low for 8 hours.

Place whole chicken carcass (skin, bones, any extra meat) and add water to the 'max' line on the stainless steel pot with filtered water. Add the salt.

Place lid on and adjust valve to 'seal'. Set Instant Pot to high pressure, 90 minutes. Instant pot will come to pressure and then turn off on its own. After cooking, allow pressure to release naturally, this can take up to 30 minutes.

Remove lid and allow stock to cool a bit, so it is not so dangerous to pour. Remove meat, bones, and cartilage (save for another batch of stock or eat).

Pour broth into jars using a funnel. Store stock in the refrigerator for up to 3 weeks.

BENEFITS OF BROTH:

Not only does broth give us something to replace our hot drinks with in the winter, but it also provides a super easy source of amino acids, healthy fats, and a vehicle for needed electrolytes (salt).

Broth is easy and inexpensive to make. We made beef broth at the start of this week and now we prep chicken broth using the leftovers from our rotisserie chicken today.

If you drink broth and then notice that you have a weird reaction, you may be having a histamine reaction to your broth. This can be solved by shortening the cooking time, preferably by using an Instant Pot. Different people have different histamine tolerances, and a histamine intolerances can be resolved as gut health is improved.

Signs of a histamine intolerance:

- Rashes including hives
- Headaches
- Nasal congestion or drip
- Persistent cough
- Digestive issues

CARNIVORE MEAT, EGG, AND DAIRY

SUNDAY
- **B** BREAKFAST SANDWICH, BUTTER COFFEE
- **L** SLICED HEART AND WHITE CHEDDAR
- **D** SCOTCH EGGS AND SOUR CREAM *PREP LIVER PATE*

MONDAY
- **B** SCRAMBLED EGGS AND CREAM
- **L** PORK RIND NACHOS
- **D** CHEESEBURGERS WITH BACON *PREP ROAST & YOGURT*

TUESDAY
- **B** HALF AND HALF YOGURT
- **L** TURKEY AND CHEESE ROLL UPS
- **D** SCOTCH EGGS AND SOUR CREAM

WEDNESDAY
- **B** SCRAMBLED EGGS
- **L** BACON-WRAPPED SCALLOPS
- **D** STEAK TOPPED WITH BUTTER AND AN EGG

THURSDAY
- **B** MILK AND EGG YOLK 'MILKSHAKE'
- **L** SHREDDED MEAT AND LIVER PATE
- **D** STEAK AND BUTTER

FRIDAY
- **B** TONGUE AND EGGS
- **L** EGG SALAD WITH SOUR CREAM
- **D** CARNIVORE PIZZA

SATURDAY
- **B** BACON
- **L** STEAK, AND A FRIED EGG WITH CHEESE
- **D** ROTISSERIE CHICKEN, SHREDDED WITH SOUR CREAM

MEAL PLAN

GROCERY List

- ☐ Beef, ground, 1/2 lb
- ☐ Beef, heart, 6 oz cooked (or sub cold cuts)
- ☐ Beef, brisket or tritip, 3-4 lbs
- ☐ Beef, ribeye, 8 oz
- ☐ Beef, strip steak, 8 oz
- ☐ Beef, tongue, 1 ea (2-3 lbs)
- ☐ Beef, marrow bones, 12
- ☐ Pork, ground, 1-1/2 lbs
- ☐ Bacon, 1-2 lbs,
- ☐ Liver pate, optional, 1 oz
- ☐ Turkey, lunch meat, 1/2 lb
- ☐ Scallops, 8 large
- ☐ Chicken, rotisserie, 1
- ☐ Butter, 1 lb
- ☐ Eggs, 2 doz
- ☐ Pork rinds, 2 bags (2-3 oz ea)
- ☐ Cheese, cheddar, 8 oz
- ☐ Sour cream, 16 oz
- ☐ Heavy cream, 1 quart
- ☐ Half and half, 2 quarts
- ☐ Yogurt, plain, 2 oz
- ☐ String cheese, 3 oz
- ☐ Milk, whole, 1 cup
- ☐ Cream Cheese, 8 oz
- ☐ Parmesan, 1/2 cup
- ☐ Sea Salt

Breakfast Sandwich, Butter Coffee

Butter coffee! If you're just starting to add dairy to your diet, you're going to love this treat of a breakfast drink! Want cheese on your breakfast sandwich without adding extra calories for today? Steal an ounce from lunch's sliced cheddar :)

For the coffee:
1 mug black coffee
1 teaspoon butter

For the breakfast sandwich:
4 ounces ground pork
1 egg
1 teaspoon butter

For the coffee, blend hot black coffee with butter in a blender or with an immersion blender for a frothy breakfast. For a fast fat boost, just stir the butter in the coffee.

For the breakfast sandwich, form ground pork into 2 large flat patties and sprinkle with sea salt.

Heat a skillet or griddle over medium heat and grease with fat. Once hot, form meat mixture into patties and fry until no longer pink in the center. Set sausage patties aside.

Add more fat if needed, and fry one egg so that the white is set and the yolk is still runny. Sandwich fried egg between two cooked sausage patties and enjoy.

> Nutrition in breakfast sandwich and butter coffee: 495 calories, 1 g carb, 43 g fat, 25 g protein

Sliced Heart and White Cheddar

3 ounces white cheddar
4 ounces beef heart

Heart is good cold, but if you don't have any cooked up yet (see page 37 for recipe), any cold cut can be used in its place.

> Nutrition above: 460 calories, 0 g carb, 32 g fat, 41 g protein

Scotch Eggs and Sour Cream

1 Scotch Egg (recipe next page)
1/4 cup sour cream for dipping

> Nutrition in Scotch Egg and Sour Cream: 602 calories, 3 g carb, 50 g fat, 32 g protein

> Day Total:
> 1557 calories, 4 g carb, 125g fat, 98 g protein
>
> 1% calories from carb, 26% calories from protein, 73% calories from fat

Scotch Eggs

4 eggs, soft boiled
1 pound pork sausage
2 cups pork rinds

Cook your eggs to desired doneness. (directions on page 48 if needed)

Crush pork rinds by placing in a heavy duty zip-top bag and crushing well with a rolling pin or whir in a food processor.

After the eggs have chilled, divide pork sausage into 8 even pieces. To cover each egg, carefully flatten one piece of the divided pork sausage into a round about the size of your palm. Do the same with a second piece of pork sausage. Place one round in the palm of your hand, then place the egg in the middle. Place the second round on top, and gently press the two rounds together until well covering every part of the egg, making sure to firmly but gently press together all seams. Repeat with the remaining eggs and sausage.

Place crushed pork rinds in a soup bowl or shallow dish and roll sausage-covered eggs in the pork rinds. Again, with your hands, firmly but carefully press pork rinds into the sausage mixture, so it evenly coats the egg.

Preheat oven to 400* F. Place Scotch Eggs on a baking sheet and bake for 25 minutes, turning once to prevent the bottoms from getting soggy.

Serve immediately or keep at room temperature for 2-3 hours before serving (as in packing for lunch).

* For Air Fryer cooking instructions see page 37.
* This recipe has a complementary video on YouTube

Bonus recipe: Pork and Parmesan Meatballs

2 pounds ground pork
1 cup shredded parmesan cheese
2 eggs (optional)
1 teaspoon sea salt

Mix together the ground pork, parmesan cheese, and optional eggs. The cheese has plenty of salt, but you may want to cook a bit of the meat mixture in a pan on the stove and adjust the salt if needed - add 1 teaspoon of sea salt at a time until you get the saltiness that you like.

Preheat broiler to high. Raise rack to the second slot down from the top in the oven. Line a metal baking tray with shallow sides (like a jelly roll pan) with parchment paper.

As the oven heats, roll meatballs into desired size (I like smaller acorn-sized meatballs) and place on the lined baking sheet; touching but not overlapping. Make sure your meatballs are all the same size so that they cook evenly.

Once preheated, broil the meatballs for 5 minutes, or until tops start to darken. If you are freezing the meatballs, remove them now and cool, then transfer to a freezer bag. Reheat/finish cooking from thawed, 350* for 20-25 minutes or until cooked through.

Move meatballs to the middle of the oven and turn the oven to 'bake' and 350* and bake for an additional 15-20 minutes, depending on how big your meatballs are.

To check doneness, cut meatball in half. Slight pink in the middle is okay, as they will continue cooking as they cool.

Serve your meatballs, topping with more cheese or cream sauce as desired.

PREPARE LIVER PATE

If you don't have pre-made liver pate, you may wish to make it today. See page 52 for recipe.

Scrambled Eggs and Cream

1 tablespoon butter
3 eggs
2 tablespoons heavy cream
1/4 teaspoon sea salt

In a medium skillet, melt butter over medium heat. As skillet heats, use a fork or whisk to whisk eggs and cream. Scramble eggs until just before set, then remove from heat and sprinkle with sea salt. Enjoy!

Nutrition: in Scrambled Eggs: 333 calories, 2 g carb, 26 g fat, 19 g protein

Pork Rind Nachos

This meal has all sorts of varieties. Here we use cheddar and liver pate, but if liver isn't your thing, substitute cream cheese.

1 ounce (about 1-1/2 cups) pork rinds
2 ounces diced beef heart
1 ounce cheddar
1 ounce Chicken Liver Pate (optional)

Place pork rinds or cracklins in an oven-proof bowl. Top with heart and sprinkle with shredded cheddar. Bake at 400* until cheddar melts. Alternatively, microwave for 1

Nutrition in whole recipe of Pork Rind Nachos: 534 calories, 3 g carb, 40 g fat, 40 g protein

minute. Top with liver pate and enjoy your nachos!

This is the perfect craving-busting food. Remember this meal for when you're tempted to go off carnivore during a stressful day or when you walk in the door absolutely famished!

Cheeseburgers with Bacon

2 pieces bacon
1/2 pound ground beef
1.5 ounce cheddar cheese

In a skillet over medium heat, fry bacon. Remove the bacon once slightly under-done (it will continue cooking as it cools), leaving grease in the pan. Use the bacon grease to fry the burgers.

To fry burgers, heat skillet up to medium-high and then sear burgers on the first side. Flip, and lower heat to medium-low to cook the other side. Add cheese continue cooking through to desired doneness.

Top burgers with cooked bacon, or chop up bacon for 'bacon sprinkles'.

Nutrition in full recipe (1 large or two medium cheeseburgers):
650 calories, 1 g carb, 45 g fat, 63 g protein

Day Total:
1517 calories, 6 g carb, 111 g fat, 122 g protein

2% calories from carb, 32% calories from protein, 66% calories from fat

Brisket or Tritip Roast

Making a roast at the beginning of the week gives you access to fast food without cooking all week long.

Tritip and Brisket are both less expensive cuts that contain lots of the yummy fat that we need for energy and to feel our best. Pop one in the Instant Pot or slow cooker and then shred with a fork and individually portion out 8-12 ounces (depending on your nutrient needs).

When I portion out my roasts, I use glass freezer containers (see what I use on the Resource Page), and add 1 tablespoon tallow and a generous helping of sea salt to the roast before freezing. Then if I'm going to be out of the house for the day or out of town for the weekend, I can just grab 1-4 of my 'carnivore freezer meals' and stick with carnivore easily no matter where I am.

To reheat, I most often use a microwave. If microwaving isn't your thing, you can thaw and then pan-fry thawed shredded roast in a skillet over medium-high heat.

This roast isn't counted as a meal today, so feel free to cook it over night and portion out in the morning.

3-4 pound brisket or tritip roast
1 teaspoon sea salt
1 cup water

Instant Pot: Place roast in the Instant Pot, add water around the roast, and sprinkle with sea salt. Cook on high pressure for 90 minutes and then let pressure release naturally (another 45 minutes or so).

Slow cooker: Place roast in a medium slow cooker, add water around the roast, and sprinkle with sea salt. Cook on low for 8-10 hours.

Half and Half Yogurt

Yogurt! This fermented dairy is delightfully mainstream. Here we make it with half and half, this not only makes it taste more mild, but it provides needed fat and less carb. When we culture at a low temperature for 24 hours, we use up the most lactose possible, and thus lowering the carb count. Where do the carb go? The cultures eat it!

*If you have **raw milk**, that's even better. It's recommended to use a room-temp-culture method like filmjolk so that you don't have to heat your raw milk and destroy the fragile enzymes.*

½ gallon (2 quarts) half and half, preferably organic
1 quart heavy cream (optional)
2 tablespoons unflavored yogurt with live active cultures to use as a starter

In a stock pot, heat half-and-half gently on medium heat, stirring approximately every 10 minutes, until milk is close to a boil. Cover, remove from burner, and allow to cool until the yogurt is comfortable to the touch, 90-110* F.

Make sure the half-and-half is not too hot at this stage, or you will kill the good bacteria that are going to make your yogurt into milk. Place yogurt starter in the warm half and half and whisk or stir to distribute evenly.

Pour milk with starter into the glass jars. Now we need to incubate, also called culture, at a consistently warm (but not too warm) temperature so that our little bit of starter eats up our lactose and multiplies all the tangy delicious beneficial strains.

Dehydrator Method: If you're using quart sized jars, they do fit in the 5-tray dehydrator you just have to tilt them to get them in there. Alternatively, place the lid back on the stockpot you used to heat the milk, and place the whole pot in the dehydrator.

Screw on lids, and shake to distribute culture even more. Place covered jars in the dehydrator, and turn to 100 degrees for a full 24 hours.

(Yogurt, Continued)

Cooler Method: Before starting your yogurt, bring a cooler into the house and open it to warm it up. A medium-to-small cooler is perfect, you need to be able to hold your yogurt and a gallon or two of hot water in containers.

After your milk and starter has been poured into glass jars, stack them in the cooler. Use hot tap water to fill 2 gallon containers (I use milk cartons) with hot water. Nestle those next to your warm yogurt warm in the cooler. Fill any excess space with a towel - it doesn't need to be tightly packed but the cooler should be full. Close the cooler and allow to incubate for 24 hours, changing out the hot water with fresh hot tap water every 6-8 hours.

Instant Pot Method: Follow the directions for your Instant Pot's model and set the culture time to 24 hours.

For most Instant Pots that have a Yogurt function the directions are like this:

- Pour milk in the instant pot. Use yogurt function and set to 'boil'. Instant Pot will turn off when it is done with this function.
- Allow milk to cool until it is comfortable to touch, but not cold.
- Add starter and whisk in well.
- Place lid on the Instant Pot and set again to Yogurt, but this time you set to 24:00 once the option for changing the time populates. IP will beep when done.

Any method: After culturing for 24-36 hours yogurt is now done and should be kept in the refrigerator.

* This recipe has a complementary video on YouTube

Nutrition per cup of half-and-half yogurt:
315 calories, 28 g fat, 5 g carb, 7 g protein

Roasted Beef Marrow Bones

Roasted marrow is the creamy custard of the carnivore world. Bone marrow contains adiponectin, which is found to have protective effects for bone health and the whole body. Adiponectin is correlated with increased insulin sensitivity (this is a good thing!), fat loss, and even has been linked with reduced risk of heart disease, diabetes, and obesity-related cancers.

Next time you throw your dog a bone, go ahead and roast some for yourself as well!

12 marrow bones
Sea salt to taste

Line a baking sheet with parchment paper. Preheat oven to 450*F. Place bones upright on baking sheet. Bake for 15 minutes, and allow to cool a bit and sprinkle with sea salt before eating. Eat marrow right out of the bone with a spoon.

Didn't eat them all? Make marrow bones into stock.

Marrow bones can be found on the Carnivore Resource Page and often at your local butcher!

Nutrition from this bonus recipe is not included in the above day total.

Source for bone marrow nutrition claims: https://www.sciencedaily.com/releases/2014/07/140703125216.htm

Nutrition per tablespoon of baked marrow:
126 calories, 12 g fat, 0 g carb, 1 g protein

Half and Half Yogurt

Tangy, refreshing, and easy, scoop some yogurt out and enjoy this morning! If you didn't make your own yogurt, choose full-fat yogurt from the store. It's harder to find but worth it for the satiety that higher fat yogurt brings.

Nutrition in 1.25 cups half-and-half yogurt: 394 calories, 6 g carb, 35 g fat, 9 g protein

Turkey and Cheese Roll Ups

Such a simple lunch, and so filling and portable! When choosing lunch meat, check ingredients carefully and choose the highest quality you can.

String cheese is commonly thought to be processed cheese, but in reality it's just mozzarella sticks. For a packaged food, it is pretty clean and nothing like the American pseudo-cheese that you may have grown up on!

3 ounces string cheese
6 ounces Applegate turkey lunchmeat

Lay out 1-2 slices of lunchmeat and roll up a cheese stick into each. Switch it up by using different kind of cheese sticks: Cheddar, Pepper Jack, etc.

This meal is easy to throw in your lunch bag - just grab a package of lunchmeat and a few cheese sticks and unwrap when you're ready to eat.

Nutrition for full recipe of Turkey and Cheese Roll Ups: 500 calories, 3 g carb, 23 g fat, 38 g protein

Scotch Egg and Sour Cream

1 Scotch Egg
1/4 cup sour cream

Nutrition in Scotch Egg and Sour Cream: 602 calories, 3 g carb, 50 g fat, 32 g protein

A1/A2 DAIRY

Think dairy isn't agreeing with you? It may be the type of cow that's making the milk. Milk from cows that have the A1 beta casein (primarily Holstein, which is where most dairy in the US comes from) gene causes digestive trouble in more people than milk from cows that are A2. If you've found that goat milk doesn't affect you, but cow milk does, it may be the type of cow.

Before you throw out the idea of ever having sharp cheddar, or delicious heavy cream again, take care to source milk from Jersey, Guernsey, or Asian cattle, which have A2 protein.

Sources:
https://www.ncbi.nlm.nih.gov/pubmed/26404362
http://cdrf.org/2017/02/09/a2-milk-facts/

Day Total:
1539 calories, 3 g protein, 106 g fat, 143 g protein 1% calories from carb, 37% calories from protein, 62% calories from fat

Scrambled Eggs

Fast and easy! You can make eggs with cheese and clean up in less time than it would take to pull through a drive through! Your body will thank you for making this choice to put a little effort into breakfast this morning as well.

5 eggs, or 3 eggs and 1.5 ounces cheddar
1 teaspoon bacon grease or other fat
Sea salt to taste

In a medium skillet, melt bacon grease over medium heat. As skillet heats, use a fork or whisk to whisk eggs. Scramble eggs until just before set, then remove from heat and sprinkle with sea salt. Enjoy!

Nutrition in full recipe:
455 calories, 2 g carb, 35 g fat, 30 g protein

Steak with an Egg and Butter

Simple and efficient is the name of the game with this meal.

1 tablespoon butter
8 ounces ribeye steak
1 egg

Melt butter in a skillet and cook steak. For specifics on the many different ways to cook steak, see page 31. As steak rests, fry egg in leftover drippings and tallow until white is cooked but yolk is still runny.

Top steak with egg and any left over butter/meat drippings from pan and enjoy!

Nutrition for all of the above: 792 calories, 0 g carb, 79 g fat, 44 g protein

Bacon-Wrapped Scallops

These are like candy on the carnivore diet! So good, and they cook quickly in the oven. For packing lunch, they can be kept warm in a thermos.

8 large sea scallops
4 slices thin bacon (Applegate or ButcherBox bacon are good thickenesses)

Preheat oven to 425*F and line a baking sheet with parchment paper. Cut bacon in half crosswise. Precook bacon for 3-4 minutes flat on the parchment. As the bacon cooks, pat scallops dry with paper towels and set aside.

Once bacon has cooled until it's cool enough to touch, wrap bacon around each scallop and secure with a toothpick.

Place on baking sheet, and repeat with the remaining scallops. Bake for 12 minutes and then serve warm.

Nutrition for above: 422 calories, 2 g carb, 31 g fat, 35 g protein

Day Total:
1669 calories, 4 g carb, 145 g fat, 109 g protein

1% calories from carb 25% calories from protein 74% calories from fat

Shredded Meat and Cream Cheese

Not a cream cheese fan? Add sour cream in place of the cream cheese or even cod liver (it's good, I promise!) for a vitamin boost. Find canned raw wild-caught cod liver in its own oil on the Carnivore Resource Page.

1 tablespoon salted butter
8 ounces brisket, shredded (from Monday's prep)
1 ounce cream cheese

In a skillet, or in the microwave, heat the shredded brisket. Add butter and cream cheese and enjoy!

> Nutrition for Shredded Meat and Cream Cheese as above: 826 calories, 2 g carb, 69 g fat, 47 g protein

Milk and Egg Yolk 'Milkshake'

The self-admittedly bizarre breakfast of Marilyn Monroe consisted of 2 raw eggs whipped into warm milk. Here we adapt the blonde bombshell's breakfast to omit the egg whites as they inhibit biotin absorption and just include the yolks.

1 cup whole milk (preferably raw)
2 egg yolks

Heat milk if desired, and whip in egg yolks using an immersion blender or stir in with a fork. Enjoy!

Nervous about raw eggs? Wash the shell before cracking, and make sure your eggs are from healthy chickens. You could also just have milk and hard-cooked eggs and call it good.

If you're using raw milk, don't heat it higher than is comfortable to touch (about 115 degrees) - this ensures the enzymes stay intact.

> Nutrition for 1 cup whole milk and 2 egg yolks: 269 calories, 13 g carb, 18 g fat, 14 g protein

> **MIND YOUR SALT!**
> It's common during the first 30-90 days of the carnivore diet to need to eat more salt than usual, even if you've previously been on keto. If you're feeling sluggish, or dehydrated, see how you feel after eating 1/4 teaspoon salt (plain) and then chugging a big glass of water. 9/10 times you'll feel much better within 10 minutes!

Carnivore Tacos

Cheese baked on parchment makes a surprisingly good taco shell!

6 ounces shredded tongue, or other ground meat
3 ounces white cheddar cheese, grated

For the cheese taco shells: Preheat oven to 350* F
Line a baking sheet with parchment paper.
Make 3 little circular piles of cheese that are about 3" across on the parchment . Leave lots of space between for the cheese to melt.

Bake for 10-12 minutes, or until edges start to turn dark and the cheese is still very melty in the middle. If you have a standard oven (not convection) rotate trays half way through to evenly cook the cheese.
Allow to cool on the cookie sheet for 5 minutes, the cheese will set.

For the taco meat: Use a knife to finely chop tongue meat if using tongue. For other ground meat, brown ground beef in a skillet over medium heat as the cheese shells cook and cool.

Once shells have cooled, fill with taco meat and enjoy!
Add sour cream if desired.

Nutrition for tacos made with tongue (whole recipe): 812 calories, 0 g carb, 65 g fat, 54 g protein

Beef Tongue

Tender, inexpensive, and available at most butchers or online, beef tongue is a surprisingly easy and tender meat. A favorite of young children, once you start making tongue you will make it on a regular basis. Plus, it's a great way to reinforce the farm-to-tableness of food and instill gratitude for our meat- this meat looks exactly how you'd expect!

1 beef tongue
Sea salt
Filtered water to cover

Slow Cooker Directions: Thaw beef tongue but do not peel. Place in slow cooker and sprinkle with 1/2 teaspoon sea salt. Cover with filtered water until the water covers the tongue by about 1/2 inch. Cook on low for 8-10 hours.

Instant Pot: Follow same directions but cook on high pressure for 90 minutes.

Remove tongue from the water and allow to cool on a cutting board. Peel off exterior and chop muscle meat into bite-sized pieces.

Nutrition for 4 ounces beef tongue: 253 calories, 0 g carb, 18 g fat, 17 g protein

Day Total:
1907 calories, 16 g carb, 152 g fat, 115 g protein 4% calories from carb, 25% calories from protein 75% calories from fat

Leftover Meat and Eggs

2 ounces tongue or leftover roast
3 eggs, fried

Nutrition for 2 ounces tongue and 3 fried eggs: 335 calories, 1 g carb, 22 g fat, 29 g protein

Egg Salad made with Sour Cream

Sour cream, or your homemade half and half yogurt make a creamy egg salad. Celery seed and pickle add flavor, but are completely optional.

4 hard boiled eggs
1/4 cup sour cream
1/4 teaspoons sea salt

Chop hard boiled eggs and mix in sour cream and sea salt.

Optional additions:

- 1 naturally fermented pickle, diced
- 1/4 teaspoon celery seed
- pinch black pepper

Nutrition for full recipe: 372 calories, 3 g carb, 27 g fat, 24 g protein

Carnivore Meatza

Pizza! Who doesn't love pizza? Pizza Friday is a low-key holiday in our house. Build your own pizza night is not only a favorite for my kids, but it's also a really fun way to entertain. Here we make our base out of ground beef, then top with cheese and a layer of pepperoni.

3/4 pounds ground beef
1 ounce pepperoni
4 ounces mozzarella
Sea salt to taste

Preheat oven to 375*F. Line a cookie sheet with parchment paper. Mix about 1/2 teaspoon sea salt into ground beef (to taste) and press ground beef into a pizza shape. Top with shredded mozzarella and sliced pepperoni. Bake for 20-30 minutes, depending on the thickness of the meat. Cut into wedges and serve.

Optional Pizza Toppings:

- Pesto or red sauce
- Sliced mushrooms (a fungi, not really a plant)
- Crushed garlic
- Crumbled sausage
- Bacon sprinkles (aka bacon bits)
- Extra cheese!

Nutrition:
927 calories, 0 g carb, 58 g fat, 95 g protein

Day Total:
1634 calories, 4 g carb, 107 g fat, 148 g protein

1% calories from carb, 61% calories from fat, 38% calories from protein

Fathead Mozzarella Dough

This dough is a perfect base for SO many things. Wrap it around hot dogs for pigs in a blanket. Use it as your pizza crust. Cut into squares and cook it til crisp for crackers. This dough is addictive and amazing!

1-3/4 cups low-moisture (not fresh) mozzarella cheese
3/4 cup ground up pork rinds
2 tablespoons cream cheese
1 egg

Pre-heat oven to 400* F.

In a medium microwave-safe bowl, place the shredded mozzarella, ground pork rinds, and cream cheese. No need to mix yet.

Microwave on high for 1 minute, stir to start combining and eliminate any hot spots (it'll come together more in later steps) and microwave for an additional 60-90 seconds.

Stir again for a few seconds, and as soon as the dough isn't scalding hot, crack the egg into it. Mix immediately, kneading like bread dough.

Once the egg is completely mixed in, the dough should be elastic, like wheat dough.
Roll into desired shape for pizza between two sheets of parchment paper. Remove top sheet and place pizza dough (keeping it on the bottom sheet of parchment) onto a baking sheet.
Bake for 20 minutes.

Once the pizza is baked, flip over (this helps the crust to hold its shape under the toppings) and top as desired. Return to oven for another 5-10 minutes to melt the cheese.

Cheese Crackers

These savory crisps are delicious topped with liver, or just on their own. They are easy to pop in the oven as you're finishing up dinner prep. Don't want to make your own? You can find Parmesan crisps pre-made in many grocery stores!

Ingredient:
1/2 cup Parmesan cheese

Preheat oven to 425* F, and preheat stoneware baking sheet if you are using stoneware. A metal baking sheet can be used as well, no need to preheat.

Grate Parmesan cheese until you have about 1/2 cup. Line a baking sheet with parchment paper.
Drop heaping teaspoonfulls of grated cheese in pile on the parchment paper, about 2-3 inches a part (it will spread).

Bake in preheated oven for 5-10 minutes, checking often. Crisps are done when they start to turn golden brown. Remove crisps from the oven and allow to cool on the parchment paper. I like to take the parchment off the baking sheet and put it right on the cool counter top to speed this process up.
* This recipe has a complementary video on YouTube

Nutrition in approx 1/6 (1 ounce before cooking) cracker recipe: 122 calories, 0 g carb, 8 g fat, 11 g protein

Baked Bacon

1 pound bacon (4 pieces for today)

Preheat oven to 350* F. Lay out 1 pound bacon on a baking sheet, sides can be slightly overlapping as they will shrink by about 20%.
Bake for 15 minutes, and check every 5 minutes after that until desired doneness.
Drain on paper towels.
Once slightly cool, but still melted, pour fat in a mason jar to use for cooking.

Nutrition in 4 pieces bacon:
160 calories, 2 g carb, 14 g fat, 10 g protein

Rotisserie Chicken with Sour Cream

Dipping rotisserie chicken in sour cream is an easy meal to have on the go. Purchase probiotic whole fat sour cream (Nancys and Tillamok both make this) for a probiotic and fat boost!

3 ounces white meat
12 oz dark meat
1/4 cup sour cream
sea salt to taste

Nutrition in approx 1/2 rotisserie chicken (mostly dark meat) with sour cream: 820 calories, 2 g carb, 51 g fat, 84 g protein

Steak, Fried Egg and Bacon

1 piece bacon
1 fried egg
8 ounces strip steak

Cook bacon in a cast iron skillet over medium heat, remove while still slightly soft. Raise heat to medium high and sear steak. Once the first side is seared, flip, and lower heat to medium-low. Continue cooking for 5 minutes, or to desired doneness. Fry egg as the steak rests, and re-heat bacon as the egg fries in the same pan. .

Nutrition for 8 ounce steak, egg, and bacon: 590 calories, 0 g carb, 41 g fat, 52 g protein

TOUGH STEAKS AND THE INSTANT POT:

If you're going to try doing a steak in the Instant Pot (Directions on page 31), strip steak or flat iron are great steaks to start with. Instant Potting this steak ensures the connective tissue is soft and easy to eat. Covering with a glistening fried egg and crisp bacon can help the less-than-beautiful presentation of an Instant Pot steak.

Day Total:
1570 calories, 4 g carb, 106 g fat, 146 g protein

1% calories from carb, 61% calories from fat, 38% calories from protein

CARNIVORE — MEAT, EGGS, DAIRY & SEASONINGS

SUNDAY
- **B** FRIED EGGS WITH CHEESE
- **L** PORK RIND NACHOS
- **D** CARNIVORE LASAGNA

MONDAY
- **B** POACHED EGGS
- **L** LEFTOVER LASAGNA
- **D** LEMON CHICKEN SOUP WITH FETA AND CHIVES

TUESDAY
- **B** BREAKFAST SOUP
- **L** PEPPERONI AND CHEESE MINI PIZZAS
- **D** BACON CHEESEBURGER CASSEROLE

WEDNESDAY
- **B** STEAK
- **L** LEFTOVER CHEESEBURGER CASSEROLE
- **D** CRACK CHICKEN (MAKE RANCH)

THURSDAY
- **B** BREAKFAST SAUSAGE
- **L** STEAK WITH BUTTER AND HOT SAUCE
- **D** LEFTOVER CRACK CHICKEN AND PORK RINDS

FRIDAY
- **B** FRIED EGGS WITH BACON SPRINKLES
- **L** JERKY AND CREAM CHEESE
- **D** ROAST BEEF IN THE SLOW COOKER OR IP WITH RANCH

SATURDAY
- **B** BREAKFAST SANDWICH
- **L** LEFTOVER SAUSAGE OR ROAST BEEF
- **D** GARLIC-PARMESAN CHICKEN WITH MUSHROOMS

MEAL PLAN

GROCERY List

Pork, ground, 3 lbs
Pork rinds, 2 packages
Bacon, 2 lbs
Chicken thighs, bone-in
  6 lbs
Chicken drumsticks, 2 lbs
Chicken, boneless thighs
  2 lbs
Beef, ground, 5 lbs
Beef, brisket or tritip, 4
  lbs
Pepperoni, 4 oz
Beef roast, any, 3 lbs

Butter, 2 lbs
Eggs, 1 doz
Cheddar, 8 oz
Cream Cheese, 24 oz
Cottage cheese, 1 cup
Feta cheese, 2 oz
Mozzarella cheese 8 oz
Parmesan cheese, 1 cup
Sour cream, 16 oz
Heavy Cream, 1 cup

Sea Salt
Garlic, 2 heads
Red sauce, 1/2 cup
Lemon, 2
Red pepper flakes
Black pepper
Chives, 1 bunch fresh
Ginger, 1 root
Mustard
Dried Chives
Dried Parsley
Onion flakes
Sage
Fennel
Ground coriander
Hot sauce
Honey, 2 tbs
No-sugar ketchup, 1/4 cup
Apple cider vinegar
Ground ginger
Cayenne
Basil, 1 bunch fresh
Jalapeño peppers, 4

Cheese Omelet

Omelets are the creative cook's favorite weekend breakfast. If you're not feeling creative in the kitchen, a scramble is always a great fall back - just scramble fillings with the eggs and call it good!

1 tablespoon butter
3 eggs
2 tablespoons filtered water
1 ounce cheddar cheese, shredded
Optional: Crumbled sausage or bacon
Sea salt to taste

In medium-sized frying pan, heat butter until melted and then use spatula to spread it across the bottom of the pan.

As the butter heats, crack eggs into a small bowl. Add water and stir eggs until yolks are evenly distributed.

Pour egg mixture into bottom of frying pan. As egg cooks, use spatula to lift or push the edge of the eggs – just slightly – then tilt the pan so the uncooked egg on top of the omelet slides to the edge of the pan and begins to cook. Continue tilting and cooking until egg is almost cooked through, then place lid on frying pan and allow the egg to cook until done.

Place cheese in a line down the middle of the omelet, and then use your spatula to fold the two empty sides of the omelet on top of the cheese and optional sausage mixture. Allow it to cook for about 30 seconds longer and then slide onto a plate.

Pork Rind Nachos

1 ounce cream cheese
2 ounces shredded brisket or other meat
1.5 ounce medium cheddar
2 ounces 4505 Meats BBQ Pork Rinds

In a microwave-safe bowl, place pork rinds. Top with globs of cream cheese and sprinkle with shredded cheddar, and finally shredded meat. Microwave on high for 1 minute, or until cheese melts.

Broil in the oven in a broiler-proof dish (usually a metal pan is best- do not broil glass or ceramic) for 2-3 minutes to avoid the microwave.

Optional Nacho Toppings:

- Cod livers
- Sliced mushrooms (a fungi, not really a plant)
- Liver Pate
- Crumbled sausage
- Bacon sprinkles (aka bacon bits)
- Extra cheese!

Nutrition for the omelet as written: 487 calories, 1 g carb, 42 g fat, 26 g protein

Nutrition for full recipe pork rind nachos: 741 calories, 1 g carb, 57 g fat, 51 g protein

Carnivore Lasagna

This lasagna is a process to make, but the results are mind-blowingly awesome. If you need a zero-carb meal to serve company, this is another great one.

The one drawback to this dish is that it is essentially cheese, cheese, and more cheese with a hint of meat. If you're going light on the dairy, a roast may be a better fit for your Sunday dinner.

For the 'noodles'
2 large eggs
4 oz cream cheese, softened
1/4 cup Parmesan cheese, grated
1 1/4 cup mozzarella cheese, shredded
2 cloves garlic, crushed

For the other layers:
1 lb ground beef
1/2 cups Red Sauce or Pesto
1 cup cottage cheese mixed with 1 clove garlic, crushed, and
   1 teaspoon Italian seasoning
Additional 1/2 cup shredded mozzarella

To make the lasagna noodles, preheat an oven to 375*F. Line a baking sheet or 9x13" pan with parchment paper. Mix softened cream cheese, shredded mozzarella cheese, Parmesan cheese, eggs, and garlic in a mixing bowl until egg is throughly mixed in. Spread this mixture onto the parchment paper evenly, making a large rectangle. Bake for 20 minutes, until edges start to turn golden. Remove from oven and allow to cool to room temperature.

As the noodles bake and cool, brown the ground beef. After browning, add in red sauce or pesto.

Mix the cottage cheese, garlic, and Italian seasoning together.

Spray a loaf pan with cooking spray, or grease with butter. Cut 'noodle' across into 3 loaf-pan-sized noodles. Place a noodle rectangle on the bottom of the loaf pan, then top with 1/3 the meat mixture and 1/3 the cottage cheese mixture. Repeat the noodle-meat-cheese pattern, ending in cottage cheese. Top the last layer of cottage cheese with the 1/2 cup shredded mozzarella cheese.

Bake, on a cookie sheet as this tends to spill over, for 35 minutes at 375*F.

If you need to make this ahead of time, you can keep it covered in the freezer or fridge, and bake from thawed for 45 minutes at 375*F.

Nutrition for 1/4 lasagna recipe: 486 calories, 10 g carb, 34 g fat, 57 g protein, 2 g fiber

Day Total:
1714 calories, 12 g carb, 133 g fat, 134 g protein, 2 g fiber (10 g net carb)

3% calories from carb, 67% calories from fat, 30% calories from protein

Eggs Poached in Stock

1 cup beef stock
2 large eggs

In a large skillet, preferably with a lid, add broth and bring to a simmer over medium heat. Once the broth is simmering, crack one egg at a time and gently add to the broth, allowing for some space between the eggs.

Once broth returns to a simmer, lower the heat to medium-low and cover if you have a lid (clear works the best). Simmer until all the white is solid, but the yolk is still runny, just a minute or two. Remove each egg with a slotted spoon or spatula.
Sprinkle with salt and serve. Reserve broth from poaching to add to soup or drink on its own alongside the eggs.

Flavor additions:
A squeeze of lemon, sprinkle of fresh snipped chives, or splash of hot sauce all add flavor elements to this simple breakfast

Nutrition for eggs poached in stock: 243 calories, 1 g carb, 15 g fat, 23 g protein

Leftover Lasagna

Everyone knows that lasagna is better the next day, and we take full advantage with yesterday's lasagna! If you're packing this lunch, reheat at home and then pack in a thermos.

Nutrition for 1/4 the Lasagna Recipe: 486 calories, 10 g carb, 34 g fat, 57g protein, 2 g fiber

Seasoned Chicken Stock

2 pounds chicken drumsticks or wings
3 cloves garlic, peeled
1 inch ginger root, peeled
1 tablespoon sea salt

Instant Pot Directions: Place all ingredients in the Instant Pot and add water to the 'max' line on the stainless steel pot with filtered water.
Place lid on and adjust valve to 'seal'. Set Instant Pot to high pressure, 90 minutes. Instant pot will come to pressure and then turn off on its own. After cooking, allow pressure to release naturally, this can take up to 30 minutes.

Slow Cooker Directions: Place all ingredients into a slow cooker, cover to 1 inch below the rim with filtered water and cover with the lid. Cook on low for 8-12 hours.

Stovetop Directions: Place all ingredients into a large stock pot, cover to 1 inch below the rim with filtered water. Simmer for 3-8 hours with a lid on.

Continue for any method: Remove lid and allow stock to cool a bit, so it is not so dangerous to pour. Remove meat, bones, and cartilage (save for another batch of stock or eat).
Pour stock into jars using a funnel. Store stock in the refrigerator for up to 3 weeks.

Greek Lemon Chicken Soup with Feta and Chives

This lemon chicken soup is delicious, and fresh and bright with the lemon flavor. If you're avoiding nightshades you'll want to omit the red pepper flakes, and possibly the black pepper.

2 tablespoons tallow or other fat

4 cups chicken stock

2 cups water

1 lemon, juiced

1/2 teaspoon red pepper flakes

1 tablespoon sea salt

1/2 teaspoon black pepper

2 oz feta cheese

6 cloves garlic

1 bunch chives, chopped

3 pounds boneless chicken thighs

In the bottom of a stock pot or using the saute function of the Instant Pot, heat fat over medium heat and add garlic, chicken stock, filtered water, skinless chicken breast or thighs (whole, we will shred it in another step), lemon zest and juice, red pepper flakes, salt, and pepper.

Once the soup is simmering, lower heat to medium-low (or low on the Instant Pot Saute Function) and cook an additional 30 minutes, or until chicken is cooked through when pierced with a knife.

If you need the soup to be done faster, use the pressure setting on the pressure cooker- high pressure for 10 minutes with the lid on and set to Seal.

Remove the chicken and shred with 2 forks on a plate or cutting board, and return to the soup. Taste and add red pepper flakes, black pepper, or salt as desired.

To serve, ladle soup into bowls. Top with snipped chives and crumbled feta. Enjoy!

Nutrition in 1/4 recipe for Greek Lemon Chicken Soup : 672 calories, 12 g carb, 42 g fat, 66 g protein

Day Total:
1401 calories, 23 g carb, 91 g fat, 146 g protein 3 g fiber

6% calories from carb 55% calories from fat 39% calories from protein

Breakfast Soup

Soup can be made more breakfast-like by adding an egg. Here we poach it right in the broth from last night's soup, infusing the egg with flavorful lemon, chicken, and chives.

1 serving (1/4 recipe) of yesterday's soup
2 eggs

To poach the eggs, use a slotted spoon to strain broth into a large skillet or saucepan (that has a lid) and bring to a simmer over medium heat. Once the broth is simmering, crack one egg at a time and gently add to the broth, allowing for some space between the eggs. Once broth returns to a simmer, lower the heat to medium-low and cover if you have a lid (clear works the best).

Simmer until all the white is solid, but the yolk is still runny, just a minute or two. Add the remaining ingredients from the soup and continue cooking a minute or two to heat. Enjoy!

Nutrition in recipe above: 815 calories, 13 g carb, 51 g fat, 79 g protein

Pepperoni Cheese Mini Pizzas

A combination of Parmesan and mozzarella also works well for these little zero-carb pizza bites. Dip in a little marinara if you are eating pizza sauce.

If you need to pack them for lunch, they pack really well after cooling!

4 ounces pepperoni
4 ounces mozzarella cheese

Preheat oven to 350*F. Line a baking tray with parchment paper. Shred mozzarella if not pre-shredded and drop in 1-tablespoon heaps, about 2-3 inches apart. Top each mozzarella heap with 1 slice pepperoni. Bake for 7-10 minutes or until pepperoni starts to crisp and cheese starts to turn golden around the edges. Remove parchment paper from the hot pan onto a cool counter top and allow to set up for 5 minutes. Enjoy!

*This recipe has a video on YouTube!

Nutrition for mini pizza bites: 500 calories, 3 g carb, 23 g fat, 38 g protein

MIND YOUR SALT!
It's common during the first 30-90 days of the carnivore diet to need to eat more salt than usual, even if you've previously been on keto. If you're feeling sluggish, or dehydrated, see how you feel after eating 1/4 teaspoon salt (plain) and then chugging a big glass of water. 9/10 times you'll feel much better within 10 minutes!

Bacon Cheeseburger Casserole

Casseroles are the ultimate comfort food. This casserole is a favorite with my family, even those not on carnivore.

4 slices bacon
2 lbs ground beef
1/4 cup no-sugar ketchup (optional)
2 tablespoons mustard (optional)
1/2 teaspoon sea salt
3 eggs
1-1/2 cups shredded cheddar cheese
1/2 cup sour cream (optional)

In a large skillet over medium heat cook bacon until still soft, but mostly cooked. Leave the bacon grease in the skillet and brown beef in it.

Once beef is browned, mix in the optional ketchup and mustard, sea salt, and eggs.

Preheat oven to 400* F. If you're using an oven-proof skillet, you can bake the casserole right in the skillet. If not, grease a casserole dish and transfer the ground beef mixture to the casserole dish, spreading in evenly. Top with cheddar cheese. Cut the bacon into small pieces and sprinkle on top of the cheese.

Bake for 20 minutes, or until cheese is melted and bacon is crisp. Allow to stand for 5 minutes before serving with sour cream if desired.

Nutrition in 1/4 recipe casserole: 500 calories, 3 g carb, 23 g fat, 38 g protein

EXTRA FOR THE FREEZER

Bacon Cheeseburger Casserole holds up well to freezer. If you buy a big package of beef or have loads of other ground meat thawed, make one of these for tonight and another two for the freezer. Assemble the casserole in a freezer-proof dish and freeze before the second baking for 20 minutes.

To cook, thaw over 48 hours in the fridge (or 6-8 hours on the counter) and then bake from chilled for 45 minutes, or until heated through, at 350* F.

MIX UP YOUR MEATS

If you have access to wild game, this cheeseburger casserole is a great recipe for wild game. In general, venison is less fatty and will need to be mixed with ground beef or even ground pork for best results. Ground turkey or chicken can be used in place of the beef, but the fat content, and calorie content, will be lowered.

In the Bacon Cheeseburger Casserole: Mix half venison and half beef, or all elk, bison, or bear in place of the beef.

Day Total:
1828 calories, 20 g carb, 105 g fat, 172 g protein 4% calories from carb, 56 % calories from fat, 40% calories from protein

Tritip or Brisket with Butter and Garlic

4-pound cut brisket (tritip ok too)
1 cup filtered water if using the Instant Pot
1 tablespoon butter
2 cloves garlic

Instant Pot:
Sprinkle brisket with sea salt on all sides. Pour filtered water in the pot of the Instant Pot.
Place brisket fat-cap up in the Instant Pot, cutting into large pieces and stacking (keeping fat up on all pieces) if needed.
Cook at high pressure (manual) for 90 minutes and allow pressure to release naturally for at least 20 minutes, then use quick release to release the rest of the pressure.

Slow Cooker:
Sprinkle brisket with sea salt on all sides. Place fat-cap up in the slow cooker on its own (no water) and cook on low for 6-8 hours. Brisket is done when the meat around the edges is starting to be able to be shredded, but the whole roast doesn't fall apart when you pick it up with tongs.

Continue for either way of cooking:
Allow to rest for 10 minutes on the cutting board before slicing. Allow cooking liquid to set, and skim fat to use in cooking or add all the liquid to your beef stock
Cut across the grain into thin slices and top with tallow and salt if desired.

Makes 3.5 pounds cooked brisket; 7 servings of 8 ounces each

Leftover Cheeseburger Casserole

Reheat another portion of cheeseburger casserole in the microwave or oven (covered).

Bonus Recipe: Cheese Sauce

Cheese sauce is delicious over pork rinds for nachos, steak that may have been cooked a touch too long, with scallops, or even used as a dip for jerky!

8 ounces cream cheese (one block)
1-1/2 cups heavy cream
8 ounces cheddar cheese (2 cups grated cheese)

Place cream cheese and cream in a saucepan. Turn heat to medium-low and cook, stirring and scraping the bottom to prevent scorching every few minutes, until cream cheese is melted - about 7 minutes total.

As the cream cheese melts, grate the cheese.

Once the cream and cream cheese are warm, keep on medium-low heat, and add grated cheese 1 large pinch (about 1 tablespoon) at a time, stirring between each addition, until half the cheese is mixed in with the cream.

Continue cooking over medium-low heat, allowing the cheese to melt, another 3 minutes. Next, add in the rest of the cheese all at once and stir gently, being sure to scrape the bottom. Turn heat to low, or turn heat off if using an electric burner that will remain hot for a few more minutes.

Allow the second half of the cheese to melt for another few minutes, or leave up to 20 minutes before serving. Give a good stir again to mix all the cheese into the sauce again before serving and enjoy!

Crack Chicken

Crack chicken is a delicious creamy ranch-flavored goodness. Directions for both the Instant Pot and Slow Cooker are provided.

4 slices thick cut bacon, diced
For the chicken:
1 tablespoon fat (tallow, chicken fat, butter)
2 pounds boneless skinless chicken breasts
1 clove garlic, crushed
Salt and fresh ground pepper, to taste
1 cup broth
For the cream cheese mixture:
8 ounces cream cheese, room temperature
2 cloves garlic, crushed
1/2 teaspoon onion powder
1/2 teaspoon dried chives

Instant Pot Directions: In the bottom of the Instant Pot, use the saute function (medium) to fry bacon. Leave grease in the bottom of the pot, and remove bacon for later. Add 1 tablespoon fat, chicken breasts, garlic, broth, salt and pepper. Cook on high pressure for 15 minutes, and allow pressure to release naturally (another 15 minutes.

Remove chicken and shred or cube. Add cream cheese, garlic, onion powder, and chives to the drippings/broth at the bottom of the Instant Pot. Simmer (saute function) and reduce until cream cheese melts and the sauce starts to thicken, about 10 minutes. Add in the shredded/cubed chicken and stir well, and then top with crumbled bacon from the first step. Enjoy!

Crack Chicken Slow Cooker Directions: Use a small slow cooker for this recipe, or shrink your slow cooker using the bowl-within-a-bowl method.

Omit the broth, and fry the bacon in a skillet and then drain grease into the slow cooker, but otherwise follow Instant pot directions. Cook on low for 8 hours, and then shred and return chicken to slow cooker with the drippings to mix in.

Nutrition for 1/4 of recipe crack Chicken:
551 calories, 3 g carb, 44 g fat, 36g protein

Bonus Recipe: Ranch Dressing

While you have most of the ingredients out already, let's whip up some ranch dressing to top your meat with.

1 cup yogurt or sour cream
1 tablespoon dried chives
1 teaspoon dried parsley
2 cloves garlic crushed
1 tablespoon dried onion flakes
Dash freshly ground black pepper
1/4 teaspoon sea salt

Blend all ingredients, adding fluid milk or cream if needed to thin, and store in the fridge. This dressing is best the next day, and best used within 1 week of making. Use it to top burgers, chicken, and more!

Breakfast Sausage

3 pounds ground pork beef, chicken, turkey, or a combination
3 teaspoon salt
1-1/2 teaspoon dried parsley
1 teaspoon dried sage
1 teaspoon ground black pepper
1/2 teaspoon fennel seeds
1/2 teaspoon crushed red pepper
1 teaspoon ground coriander
1/4 cup bacon fat for frying

In a medium mixing bowl, mix meat and all seasonings.

Optional: cover and chill over night to allow all the flavors to meld. This step isn't essential, but really helps the flavors to combine.

Heat a skillet or griddle over medium heat and grease with bacon fat or other cooking fat. Once hot, form meat mixture into patties and fry until no longer pink in the center if eating immediately, or still slightly pink if storing to reheat later.

For crumbled sausage, brown, breaking up chunks with a spatula. and then drain before storing.

* this recipe has a video on YouTube

> Recipe makes 24 patties total. Nutrition per 3 patties: 601 calories, 1 g carb, 33 g fat, 63 g protein

---

Freezer Directions:

Freeze sausage patties flat on a large metal cookie sheet, then transfer to a zip-top bag or freezer container once frozen (about 6 hours). This is called flash freezing and helps prevent the sausage patties from sticking together when they are frozen.

Freeze browned crumbled sausage in desired portion amounts (1-1/2 cups is a good amount) in freezer bags or freezer-proof containers. Use within 6 months if frozen, 7 days if refrigerated.

Brisket with Butter, Cream Cheese and Hot Sauce

Heat up roast and add butter, cream cheese, and a dash of hot sauce for easy nutrition, flavor, and health all in one little bowl.

6 ounces leftover brisket
1 teaspoon butter
1 ounce cream cheese or leftover cheese sauce
Dash hot sauce

Leftover Crack Chicken with Pork Rinds

Crack chicken is addictive and creamy on its own... adding crunchy pork rinds for dipping elevates it even further.

2 cups pork rinds, preferably Epic or 4505 brand
1 Serving Crack Chicken (yesterday)

Prepare: Jerky from a Roast

This jerky is flavorful and perfectly portable! Omit the honey/syrup if desired.

3-pound beef roast
2 tablespoons honey or maple syrup
6 cloves garlic, crushed
1/2 teaspoon black pepper
1/4 cup apple cider vinegar
1 teaspoon cayenne
1/2 teaspoon ginger
2 tablespoons sea salt

For ease of slicing, place thawed roast in freezer for 45-60 minutes; a slightly frozen roast is easier to slice. Set a timer so you don't forget- a solidly frozen roast is not easy to slice ;)

Use a sharp knife to slice roast into thin strips (1/4 inch thick or less if you can) and place strips into a freezer bag or bowl. Cover with remaining jerky ingredients and toss to coat meat evenly. Place in the fridge for 12-24 hours (covered if using a bowl), stirring or flipping the bag once half way through to evenly distribute marinade.

After marinading, place strips of meat on dehydrator tray- they can be touching but not overlapping. Dry on the highest setting your dehydrator (See the resource page for the dehydrator that I have and love) has for 7 hours. Store in the fridge or freezer.

Nutrition per 1/20th jerky recipe:
110 calories, 4 fat, 02carbs, 14 g protein

FAT BOMBS:

After a generation or two of avoiding fat, we are introducing it back into our diet with beautiful results. When we consume natural, whole-food fats our whole body benefits. Those who are eating a high-fat, low-carb diet may even struggle to consume enough calories- that's where fat bombs come in. These little pockets of delicious fat are packed with energy, essential fatty acids, and are the ideal way to consume fat-soluble vitamins.

Our skin loves the fatty acids, which help reduce aging lines and give us a youthful glow, and omega 3 fatty acids may play a role in the prevention of skin cancer. We feel full longer after eating, and have a long-lasting energy source to draw from for prolonged energy.

See a delicious fat bomb recipe on the next page.

Day Total:
1539 calories, 3 g protein, 106 g fat, 143 g protein 1% calories from carb, 37% calories from protein, 62% calories from fat

Fried Eggs with Bacon Sprinkles

2 pieces bacon
3 eggs
1/4 teaspoon sea salt

Nutrition for all of the above: 350 calories

Jerky and Cream Cheese

Softened cream cheese is a delicious dip! And jerky makes perfect meat dippers.

10 pieces beef jerky
1 ounce cream cheese

Nutrition for beef jerky and cream cheese: 433 calories, 4 g carb, 28 g fat, 41 g protein

Brisket with Ranch

Ranch is a great topping for meat, giving you flavor and creaminess.

8 ounces Roast, from Wednesday
1/4 cup ranch dressing or sour cream
1 tablespoon butter

Nutrition for 8 ounces roast with 1/4 cup ranch and butter:
520 calories, 38 g fat, 42 g protein

Bacon Jalapeño Cream Cheese Fat Bombs

These savory keto jalapeño pepper fat bombs are a snap to make and a treat to eat. To increase the healthy probiotics use organic cultured cream cheese from the dairy section of your local health food store.

8 ounces (1 cup) full fat cream cheese
4 slices bacon chopped and cooked, grease reserved
4 ounces (1/2 cup) loosely filled shredded cheddar cheese
4 jalapeño peppers stems and seeds removed
3 ounces (1/3 cup plus 1 tablespoon) tallow, melted
2 ounces (1/3 cup) bacon grease

Cook bacon over medium heat in a medium skillet. Tip: You can make 'bacon crackers' by cutting bacon into squares and then cooking- the fat bombs can then be served on top of these, or between these.

Dice Jalapeño peppers finely after removing stems and rinsing out seeds.

Combine cream cheese, cheddar cheese, diced Jalapeño, bacon grease, and melted tallow. Do not include the cooked bacon in this step or it will become soggy.

Press cream cheese mixture into a parchment-lined loaf pan and chill for 2-3 hours.

Set bacon pieces aside for serving.
Once cream cheese mixture is firm, remove from loaf pan and cut into 18 equal pieces.
Gently roll into balls and roll balls into crumbled bacon as desired. Enjoy immediately or store before covering in bacon in the fridge for 5 days or in the freezer for up to 4 weeks.

Nutrition per fat bomb (recipe makes 18): 2 fat bombs included in today's nutrient calculator: 134 calories, 13 fat, 1 carb, 3 g protein	Day Total: 1539 calories, 3 g protein, 106 g fat, 143 g protein 1% calories from carb, 37% calories from protein, 62% calories from fat

Breakfast Sandwich

2 pork breakfast sausage patties
1 fried egg
1 ounce cheddar
1 piece bacon

In a skillet over medium heat, Fry bacon, and then fry sausage patties in bacon grease. Remove bacon and sausage and fry egg in the grease, keeping the yolk runny.

Top hot sausage with cheese, then slide the fried egg on top and top with the second sausage patty.

Leftover Brisket

Leftovers are the name of the game for an easy lunch on the go. We're still eating our brisket from Wednesday, add some butter and cream cheese and garlic for a creamy topping.

1 ounce cream cheese
1 tablespoon salted butter
8 ounces shredded brisket
1 clove garlic, crushed

Pan-fry brisket in butter or heat in the microwave and top with butter, cream cheese, and crushed garlic.

Garlic-Mushroom Chicken

This Garlic-Mushroom Chicken is a favorite. It's easy to make ahead of time to pop in the oven just before dinner, and leftovers are amazing the next day as well.

1 tablespoon butter
8 chicken thighs preferably skin on bone out but any chicken thighs work
1/4 teaspoon sea salt
Pinch freshly ground black pepper

For the garlic sauce:

8 cloves garlic crushed
8 ounces bacon chopped into 1/2-inch pieces
16 ounces baby portabello mushrooms
1 cup heavy cream
4 ounces Parmesan grated (about 3/4 cup grated)
Salt to taste
1 tablespoon dried parsley

Cook the chicken:
Preheat oven to 400* F. In a large skillet, melt butter over medium-high heat. Careful, it's hot! Once skillet is pre-heated, sear the chicken for 3-4 minutes on each side, until starting to turn golden brown. You will probably have to do this in batches.

Once seared, place skin-side up in a 9×13" or similarly sized casserole dish. Once all the chicken is in the dish, sprinkle with sea salt and bake for 20 minutes if boneless, or 30 minutes for bone-in.

Mushroom Chicken Continued:

For the cream sauce:

As the chicken bakes, using the same pan that you used to sear the chicken (without draining), add crushed garlic and saute until turning fragrant and starting to brown, just a minute or two.

Add chopped bacon to the garlic and cook, stirring every minute or two, until bacon starts to crisp but is still slightly soft. While the bacon cooks, slice your mushrooms. Use a slotted spoon to remove bacon once desired doneness.

Once bacon is removed, add in mushrooms and cook in the bacon grease until soft. Once soft, add in cream and give the mushrooms a stir. By now the chicken should be nearly done, if not, just remove the cream and mushrooms from the heat.

Once chicken is done pour the cream/mushrooms over the chicken, sprinkle with Parmesan, then parsley, then reserved bacon. Return to the oven for 10 minutes to allow all the flavors to combine.

> Nutrition for 1/8 recipe (1 thigh + sauce) 417 calories, 2 g carb, 32 g fat, 26 g protein

Bonus Recipe: Garlic Herb Butter

1 pound butter, softened overnight on the counter top
4 cloves garlic
1 teaspoon sea salt
2 tablespoons snipped herbs (chives and basil)
1 lemon, zested

Use a fork or food processor to mix all ingredients together. Press into ramekins and keep one in the fridge for current use, and any extra in a freezer container for later.

Herbed butter on steak is a treat! Make some of this garlic herb butter with whatever herbs you have on hand or whatever fresh herbs look good at the store.

> Day Total:
> 1709 calories, 5 g carb, 128 g fat, 123 g protein, 1 g fiber 1% calories from carb, 30% calories from protein, 69% calories from fat

Bacon & Coffee

Many people enjoy intermittent fasting on the carnivore diet, but I often find that I'm hungry around 10. Considering I get up at 4 a.m. (by choice! I'm a morning person!) not eating until 10 may be a form of Intermittent Fasting.

On weekends, I often serve the kids a light breakfast of half-and-half yogurt with berries, and then make a bacon-and-eggs breakfast for everyone later in the morning.

A few pieces of bacon holds me over until lunch, which is often our largest meal.

You'll see the recipe for Scotch Eggs throughout this book as well; I didn't include them in my 'favorite meals' because we've already covered them, but pre-making 6-8 of them at once, and then popping them in the air fryer is another favorite breakfast of mine!

QUITTING COFFEE ON CARNIVORE:

As I was in the process of writing this book, I did finally quit coffee using the amino acid DLPA as a supplement and cutting down to one cup, then half a cup, then just plain iced tea for a few days. The calmness that I feel with the combination of carnivore without coffee is fantastic!
You, too, can quit coffee if you'd like to! It's really not that hard, and when I'm a coffee drinker it's not uncommon for me to drink a whole pot of coffee before my children wake up - I too understand the love of coffee. But like all things, it's not bad to take a break from once in a while.

Pork Rind Nachos

Pork rind nachos are a comfort food staple. The cheese is yummy and gooey, and even though I feel better not eating cheese... it still makes it into my diet plenty often.

Smoked Cod Liver can be found at the resource page at thecarnivoremealplan.com. Once you've been on carnivore for a few days, you'll realize that this is the 'dessert of meat'. Cod liver is subtly sweet and has a custard-like consistency. No wonder cod liver is a prized superfood! Drain the vitamin-rich oil into a small jar to use as a supplement - it is rich in vitamins A and D and omega 3 fatty acids.

1 ounce cream cheese
1 can smoked cod liver, drained (reserve the oil as a supplement omega 3 and vitamins A & D)
1.5 ounce sharp cheddar
2 ounces 4505 Meats BBQ Pork Rinds

In a microwave-safe bowl, place pork rinds. Top with globs of cream cheese and sprinkle with shredded cheddar, and finally shredded meat. Microwave on high for 1 minute, or until cheese melts.

Broil in the oven in a broiler-proof dish (usually a metal pan is best- do not broil glass or ceramic) for 2-3 minutes to avoid the microwave.

Nutrition for full recipe pork rind nachos: 741 calories, 1 g carb, 57 g fat, 51 g protein

Salmon Patties with Lemon Butter

(makes 4 servings)

Salmon patties are a delicious way to eat fish! Top with lemon butter for a special treat and extra fat and calories. Can also be made with tuna if desired.

Three 5 to 6-ounce cans of wild-caught salmon or 12 ounce salmon fillet
2 eggs
1/4 cup crumbled pork rinds (optional)
2-3 tablespoons ghee for frying

Canned version: Open and drain salmon by pressing cut lid on top of the salmon firmly while turning upside down over the sink.

Place salmon, eggs, and shredded coconut in a bowl and mix with a fork until egg is throughly distributed. This does not need to be a puree, but should be uniform.

Allow salmon mixture to rest (this helps the coconut to hold the mixture together) while you heat a large skillet or griddle (flat side) over medium heat.

Once skillet is pre-heated, add 1 tablespoon of fat and allow to melt. As the fat melts, form small patties out of the salmon, 'slider' size, or mini-burger size.

Once the edges start to look firm, and the top of the un-cooked patty is also starting to loose its shine a little bit, - about 5 minutes of cooking- use a thin metal spatula to carefully flip. The side that is cooked should be starting to brown.

Cook for another 3 minutes on the other side and then serve.

Fillet version: In a food processor, pulse whole raw salmon fillet (skin will probably clump up and can be removed or worked in) with the bones in and everything in a food processor. Once it's been pureed well, add in the eggs and pork rinds and pulse again to mix. Proceed, frying in ghee, as with the canned salmon patties.

For the lemon butter:

1/4 cup (1/2 stick) butter, softened but not melted
1 lemon, zested
pinch sea salt

Fold lemon zest and sea salt into butter and press lemon butter into a ramekin. Spread as desired on salmon patties, and then save the remainder covered in the ramekin.

WHOLE FISH PATTIES:

Pureeing the whole fish, bone and all, is a great way to increase calcium in the diet. Small fish bones are tedious to pick out, but dissolve easily in the food processor.

Elk Jerky

This jerky is a little more tough than you may be used to, but it's a delicious and easy source of protein! Pulse until crumbly in the food processor and add in melted fat if you want to make pemmican for a higher fat version.

2 pounds elk roast or steaks
1 tablespoon sea salt
2 tablespoons apple cider vinegar (optional)
4 cloves garlic, crushed (optional)

Mix all ingredients and allow to chill, covered, overnight. Dry in dehydrator in a single layer for 6-12 hours. Store in air-tight container in the freezer until you need to take it out. Jerky should be fine at room temp for a few days, like if you are back packing or camping.

Garlic Mushrooms

Mushrooms are a maybe food on the carnivore diet. Not a plant, but also not an animal fungi are included by some. They are delicious as a side, in scrambled eggs, or floating in stock as a soup. My favorite way to eat them is with burgers. I get a big container of baby portabello mushrooms at Costco each week and sautee them all up at once. After taking what we need for that evening, I store the rest in a covered container for use throughout the week.

This recipe takes about 30 minutes to make, but can be used all week. I like to start this as soon as I start preparing dinner so it can cook the whole time.

1/4 cup butter or bacon grease
6 cloves garlic, crushed
1 pound baby portabello mushrooms, or mushrooms of choice
1 teaspoon sea salt

In a large skillet, melt butter over medium heat. Crush garlic and add to the butter and sautee until golden. As the garlic browns, rinse and thinly slice mushrooms. If the end of the stem is blemished, just cut it off and use the rest. Add mushrooms to the garlic and butter as you slice them. Lower the heat to medium low and continue stirring as the mushrooms cook, for another 20 minutes or until completely soft and any liquid has evaporated off. Enjoy!

Deviled eggs:

Shortcut: Slice eggs in half, and dollop a bit of mayo on the top of each yolk and then squirt a bit of yellow mustard on top of the mayo. It's like a deviled egg in your mouth, without the work!

8 Hard-Cooked Eggs
¼ cup ranch dressing (page 82) or bacon mayo (page 56)
1 tablespoons prepared yellow or dijon mustard
Optional: Fresh chives, paprika, and/or crumbled bacon to garnish

Slice hard-cooked eggs in half lengthwise.
Pop out the yolks by gently applying pressure to the outside of the egg white where the yolk is.
Place yolks in a small bowl or sandwich-size zip-top bag.
Add bacon mayonnaise or homemade ranch dressing to the yolks.
If using a bowl, mash yolks with a fork. If using a zip-top bag, press out air, close, and then mash yolks with your hands (this is a great activity for kids).
Add mustard as needed to get the consistency of pudding.
Use a teaspoon to spoon yolk mixture into the indents in the egg whites. If you are using a zip-top bag, cut off the corner of the bag (just a small triangle- about an inch from the tip) and pipe into the egg whites.
Snip chives finely with scissors over the deviled eggs to garnish, and/or sprinkle with crumbled bacon.

Nutrition per 4 halves: 261 calories, 23 g fat, 13 g protein, 1 g carb.

Parmesan Baked 'Fried' Chicken

No messy frying on the stove, just pop these nuggets in the oven and you're good to go! The kids love the familiar shape, look, and texture. Dairy free? Sub pork rind crumbs for the parmesan cheese.

2 pounds boneless skinless chicken thighs (or tenders, nutrition calculated with thighs), cut into bite-sized pieces of thin strips
2 eggs
1/2 cup parmesan cheese, grated or powdered
1/4 cup crushed pork rinds (optional)
1 tablespoon dried parsley
1/2 teaspoon sea salt
1/2 teaspoon paprika (optional)
1/4 teaspoon freshly ground black pepper

Preheat oven to 375* and optional - line a baking tray (with sides) with parchment paper.

Cut chicken into bite-sized pieces and drop pieces into the two eggs in a medium bowl, mixing gently to cover.

In a shallow dish such as a pie pan, combine parmesan cheese, pork rind crumbs, parsley, sea salt, paprika, and black pepper. a few pieces of chicken at a time, remove the chicken from the egg and allow most of it to drip off, then press all sides of the chicken into the parmesan mixture.

Place parmesan-covered chicken on prepared baking dish so that it is touching but not overlapping. This will probably take up 2-3 baking dishes, or you can use the same dish and bake in batches, refrigerating the coated chicken between batches.

Bake for 25-30 minutes, or until center of the chicken is cooked and the parmesan crust turns golden brown. Serve with mustard if desired.

Vodka Soda

On a Saturday night out, a vodka soda is my drink of choice.   Vodka-soda is a sugar-free cocktail that is easily swapped out for just soda water with lime when you're done and nobody you're out with will know the difference.

1 shot vodka (or silver tequila)
1 wedge lime
Soda water, no sugar

Pour vodka over ice, cover with soda water (seltzer) and add a squeeze of lime. Garnish with a lime wedge or curl of lime zest if desired.

Alcohol on the Carnivore Diet:

Though alcohol is a toxin, and does contribute to leaky gut, some of us still choose to indulge. On carnivore (or keto!) you will feel the effects of alcohol much more than you did when you were carb fueled. Two drinks over an evening is my limit, and I drink water between too. Any more than two and suddenly my frontal cortex is numb enough that I think I should get rocky road ice cream too, and that all too often sets off a sugar spree that lasts days or more.

When you're drinking alcohol on carnivore, remember to take your salt when you get home to prevent a dehydration headache. Drink too much on accident? Activated charcoal can absorb some of it out of your stomach.

Thinking you're better off skipping the booze? Good for you! And if alcohol cravings are something you've struggled with in the past, you may be encouraged to know that being in ketosis naturally suppresses alcohol cravings. It's for that reason that keto-friendly food is often provided in top rehab centers.

TIPS FOR SUCCESS

If dieting were easy, we'd all be fit, thin, exhibiting glowing skin, and full of energy. The truth is that changing your diet takes effort! Even if the diet is as simple and straight forward as carnivore is.

For some, they will have no problem succeeding in being zero-carb for their intended duration. Others (you know who you are!) can use the following tips to maximize success.

• **Start keto first**, and make sure you have been in ketosis for at least 5 weeks. If you need help getting into ketosis, I have a Keto Family Class that is 5 weeks long and designed to get you into ketosis fast and keep you there.

• **Salt! Salt! Salt!** If you're feeling low energy, light headed, nauseous, headachy, or otherwise 'not good' take 1/2 teaspoon of salt plain, followed by a big glass of water and most of the time, your symptoms will be resolved in less than 10 minutes. If plain salt doesn't work, use 1/4 teaspoon potassium chloride (No-Salt brand salt substitute found in most grocery stores and contains potassium chloride) in addition to the sea salt.

During your first month of carnivore, your salt needs are super high! The good news is that you adjust after you adapt to carnivore, approx 30 days in for most people. After you adjust, salting your food to taste is usually plenty.

* See thecarnivoremealplan.com for a video that goes into further detail about your salt and electrolyte needs.

• **Plan 3 things to fail at** during your first 4 weeks on carnivore. Yes, we are planning on failing here! This month we are going to compromise on non-diet things in order to complete our dietary goal.

Some things you may plan on failing: Folding and putting away laundry, exercising, cooking elaborate meals for other members of your family (my family had take-and-bake pizza and a stark lack of vegetables my first week of carnivore, and we never do that!), Volunteering, home renovations (though this can be a great distraction), extra projects at work, etc. This is a temporary and effective form of self care so that you have the bandwith to complete your dietary goals.

• **Plan for self care and support for your whole self.** Self care is a hot topic lately, but it's incredibly important. Many people with chronic health issues (including, and maybe especially related to weight) are in punishment and blaming mode. Planning non-food ways to care for yourself is essential in breaking out of this negative mindset.

Self care is about healthy choices and eliminating guilt or shame as we enjoy them. Indulging in something while feeling like we are 'bad' is not self care. Nor is indulging in something that you know is harming your body and mental health (goodbye sugar and probably most alcohol!).

Think of three ways you can take care of yourself this week in the same way you would take care of a small child or friend you care about. Are you tired? Go to sleep and work on your responsibilities in the morning.

Need to rest? A binge-watching session of Netflix may be called for. Feeling antsy? A trail walk and fresh air daily may be your self care.

Have a recurring relationship, work, or emotional issue that keeps popping up? Schedule a series of therapy appointments. Often you can clear an issue in just 3-4 sessions, it's not something you have to commit to long-term unless you want to. I'm partial to EMDR-based therapy, attachment theory, and DBT.

Feeling bored or stuck in your work? Start an Audiable membership for audio books or find some podcasts that you love and indulge in these as you clean or get your fresh air! A nice mix of fiction/entertainment and nonfiction to inspire you to learn and grow.

*This is my self care of choice- I allow myself to buy unlimited audio books without guilt to listen to as I walk and run and clean, and I make sure I at least walk a 1-mile loop to get outside each day.

- **Don't insist on all organic/grassfed meat.** If your budget is tight, it can seem impossible to spend $270 on a box of organic grassfed meat from Butcherbox or your local ranch right now. After the first couple weeks on carnivore most people realize that their food spending has gone WAY down, so if you need to start with less expensive cuts of grocery store meat until your bank account reflects this saving, that is a great compromise that moves you toward your goal.

- **The most important time to succeed is immediately after you've failed.** If you 'accidentally' eat a bunch of oatmeal cookies like I did my 2nd week on the carnivore diet, hop right back on the carnivore train and eat your steak for dinner and eggs for breakfast! Just because you ate 4 (or a dozen) cookies it doesn't mean that you have to do that again tomorrow. Acknowledge that you don't feel good eating like that, and move on.

- **Keep meat on hand and thawed.** I move 2-3 days' worth of meat from my freezer to a dedicated meat thawing bowl in my fridge as soon as I'm down to my last 2-3 packages of meat. The bowl keeps the fridge clean from the inevitable package that leaks, and keeps all my food in one place. Sure, you can run to the grocery store daily and grab a ribeye or package of ground beef, but keeping plenty of meat at home and ready to go is simple to do and sets you up for success.

- **One thing at a time.** If you're one of those people constantly fails at meeting their goals, maybe your goals are too big. Get the carnivore diet down and on auto pilot, and THEN consider quitting coffee, joining the gym, or taking up a new sport. Baby steps!

TROUBLESHOOTING

You know you will thrive eating all meat, but why does it seem so difficult to do?! We're undoing a lifetime of eating a less-than-optional diet and need to reset our digestive system and ways of thinking. Most likely, especially if you start meat-based keto first, your transition to carnivore will be no problem! If you do encounter problems, look for common solutions here.

Problem: You're tired, spacey, or brain foggy.

Reason #1 Salt! You need salt! Go to thecarnivoremeailplancom and watch the salt video. It take a 8 minutes to watch it and avoid throwing out the previous days of work you've put in.

Reason #2: You're trying to intermittent fast too, or you're just not eating enough.

If you're hungry, but you're choosing to fast, it quickly uses up your impulse control. Yes, fasting is a great tool, and yes, I use it too, but when I'm doing carnivore I have a hard time sticking with only animal foods and also intermittent fasting. So, instead of sticking with both intermittent fasting and carnivore, go ahead and eat when you're hungry! Make something delicious... at 6 am one morning last week I cooked up a half pound of shrimp and a huge steak.

Problem: You're running out of money and/or meat.

Plants are cheap, there's no doubt about it. You can get the calories you need to survive for the day from sugar, soybean oil, wheat, or potatoes for just pennies. But it's surviving, not thriving. By that same logic you could live in a falling apart shack in the desert and *survive* for cheap. But that isn't a quality of life, is it?

But I know sometimes it isn't a choice - you just don't have that much money for food. So let's talk about how you can do carnivore for cheap.

Tallow! You can buy grassfed high-quality tallow for cheap. That's a whole jar of mucho calories, and they're healthy calories! Go check out even your expensive health food store - you'll probably find grassfed tallow for $6/pint. A pint has something around 4000 calories in it - it is a very inexpensive source of calories.

Lower quality beef, chicken, and pork- If you're like me, you really appreciate sustainable farming, and you do your best to source your food. When you switch to eating a human-appropriate diet (all animal foods!) this can be hard to maintain. You may have been relying on coconut products, grains, legumes, or other foods that were harming your body before starting carnivore, so you now see a spike in your grocery bill. It's okay to finish out the month on less expensive meats! Go ahead and really give carnivore a try, and eat the 99 cent/dozen eggs, 2.99/pound ground beef, .49/pound chicken thighs, and slow cook that enormous pork roast. Liver, marrow bones, and sea salt are cheap if you look around for the right sources.

The animal is doing the filtering for you, and your obligation for this month is to finish your health experiment and see how you do eating this way - you aren't obligated to single-handedly fix the entire food system. As time goes on, you can adjust your finances and lifestyle accommodate better farming practices, but for now, take the meat that's available - even if it's from Walmart (we totally have Walmart beef in our fridge right now) and finish your carnivore experiment!)

Problem: You're hungry and have cravings or you keep eating off plan 'on accident'.

Keep meat on hand, and make it easier to eat meat. If you need to buy all-beef hotdogs and pre-seasoned breakfast sausage so that you're not hungry, go do that! It's easy to 'accidentally' eat other things if you don't have meat thawed and planned for, so take a minute now to make sure you're stocked for the week and you're thawing a few days' or meat at a time.

Problem: You're overwhelmed at doing a full 30 days (or 3 months or 1 year) of Carnivore.

Shorten your goal. If you're a few days in and going all 4 weeks seems overwhelming, shorten it to 10 days. Or 7. Anything is better than nothing! Just push for a few more days, and then reflect on what you've learned!
Lots of people do this with breastfeeding when they find breastfeeding to be overwhelming (for those who haven't done it, it's a commitment of time and energy that doesn't come naturally to every mother) You can do the same thing feeding yourself - just set a small goal, and celebrate when you make it there! And you can always keep going :) This keeps the focus positive, and keeps you feeling successful.

Problem: You have sleep troubles.

Changing our microbiome quickly eliminates the out-of-balance and pathogenic fungi and bacteria rapidly and can cause temporary sleep issues. With this change, the over growth of pathogenic organisms die off. With this die off, there is a release even more of the chemicals (toxins) that they were giving off in small doses.

This can overwhelm the detoxification system and over load the pineal gland with toxins. What is the pineal gland responsible for? Melatonin production! What is melatonin? Our sleep hormone!

Magnesium and Sleep: In addition to ridding the body of pathogenic bacteria, we lose water weight on carnivore as our inflammation level goes down. This is a good thing and an overall indicator that our body is no longer producing a chronic inflammatory response. As our body sheds inflammation and the electrolytes become out of balance, we may find that we need more magnesium. Magnesium is also essential in sleep and relaxing the muscles, so supplementing with magnesium is helpful for improving sleep.

Epsom salt soaks are helpful both for magnesium (epsom salt is magnesium sulfate) and for sulfur, which is necessary for our detoxification pathways. To soak in epsom salts, add 1 cup to your bath or a foot bath and soak for at least 10 minutes. This can be done nightly.

On carnivore you will also find that you are more sensitive to caffeine and alcohol, which can also impact your sleep.

Problem: You have bathroom troubles.

There is a 5-part video series on the resource page that covers everything about poop for those who need more information than this brief overview.

First off, it's normal to have less bowel movements on the carnivore diet. There's a lot of bathroom myths to bust about how often you need to go to the bathroom to be healthy. The truth is that when you eat a diet that is made up of highly nutrient dense foods, your body can USE all that food efficiently. When our diet is high in indigestible foods and our gut is inflamed, the food passes through before we've absorbed everything from it. It's normal for carnivores to have bowel movements every 2-5 days. Usually those who eat dairy and eggs go more often than those who stick with just meat. Constipation is a problem when there is pain and straining with bowel movements, and they are hard or dry.

Sometimes, however, the opposite is a problem with the carnivore diet and you're having runny watery bowel movements This is often caused by fat malabsorption, or too many electrolytes.

Fat malabsorption is a problem especially for those who are not used to eating a high fat diet, or who have lowered stomach acid levels. Carnivore is a high fat diet, and meat is digested nearly completely in the stomach rather than the intestines. When we've been eating a low-fat high-plant-food diet, our body adjusts to lower the stomach acid strength (high stomach acid strength is low ph, it gets confusing!), produce less of it, and produce less enzymes needed to break down fats and meats. *When we're not breaking down the meat well enough to use it, it will pass through our system quickly - causing diarrhea.*

If you are on a stomach-acid blocking medication, ask your doctor about reducing the strength or eliminating it completely. Look into natural solutions to acid reflux issues. Most acid reflux issues are cleared up by the carnivore diet, but there is a transition period where your body isn't making enough stomach acid to digest your meat, and it needs to adjust. A slow transition onto the carnivore diet over 3-4 weeks usually helps this transition. Beta HCL, digestive enzymes, and apple cider vinegar all are recommended supplements for the transition. See the Carnivore Meal Plan Resource Page for more information on these supplements.

Overdoing the salt or potassium or magnesium that you take as a supplement can also cause watery bowel movements. To see if this is the case, simply eliminate or way back off on your electrolyte consumption. The phenomenon of salts causing diarrhea is called a 'salt flush' and is used to clear out the digestive tract before certain medical procedures.

Problem #7: You aren't seeing the healing you expect from Carnivore, even after 6-8 weeks of being consistent.

Reason 1: You aren't eating the correct amount. If you are feeling tired, moody, or having excessive cravings, it is very likely that you aren't eating enough calories! Do a quick spot-check and use a calorie tracker to see how many calories you eat today, and how you feel. Most women need 1400-2000 calories a day to maintain their weight, and most men need 1700-2500 depending on height, weight, and activity level. If you are far outside those ranges, no wonder you don't feel good! Eat more! :)

On the other hand, you'll also want to check your calorie consumption if you aren't losing weight that you desire to lose at a rate of 2 pounds per month. A loss of 2 pounds is a lot of weight loss!

Reason 2: You're allergic to dairy and/or eggs.

Food allergies can be pesky, with symptoms that pop up in the form of skin rashes, brain fog, digestive upset, and more. If you haven't done a 5-day break from dairy and eggs it's okay to do a braek from one at a time) and you're not seeing the healing you were hoping for on carnivore, go ahead and try going egg-free for 5 days, and then dairy-free for 5 days. Usually you'll notice a flare in symptoms upon reintroduction- this flare tells you there's an allergy.

Dairy and egg allergies are fairly common, especially for those with eczema and other skin rashes.

Reason 3: You're oxalate dumping too fast.

Oxalates... they're the sharp little compounds that combine with calcium to make up kidney stones, are linked with joint pain, fibromyalgia, and other chronic pain, and are even associated with some forms of autism. Oxalates are anti-nutrients found in leafy green vegetables and other plant food including keto favorites like cocoa, almonds, and spinach. Some people process oxalates out easily, and some people have a harder time eliminating oxalates, which causes a buildup in the body.

For those who tend to buid up oxalate, once you go on a no oxalate diet, your body may rapidly start 'dumping' out the oxalate stored in your body.

If you have increased pain anywhere including in joints, ears, throat, urinary tract, kidneys, eyes, etc consider that you may be dumping oxalates. If you have oxalate issues, you'll want to cut back on oxalate foods gradually. You also will want to do more research than this book covers. Sally Norton is considered the most knowledgeable about oxalates and I recommend reading and listening to her work.

Reason 4: You have heavy metals.

Heavy metals are destructive little molecules, attaching themselves to cell receptor sites, gumming up how organs function, contributing to leaky gut, and more. If you've eaten a modern diet, suffered from any digestive issue, consumed antibiotics or pharmacuticals, it's likely that you have a buildup of heavy metals in your body.

When the detoxification system slows down its function, or you're exposed to an excessive amount of heavy metals, your body becomes overloaded. Even 'sub toxic' (amounts lower than would show up as toxic on a heavy metals test) amounts of metals like mercury, lead, cadmium and arsenic, all notably cause problems in the body's bodily functions. Hormone receptor sites become blocked, nerves don't receive their signals, and as a protective measure, overgrowth of Candida accumulates to protect the body from mercury.

If you have chronic health problems despite a squeaky-clean diet, addressing the metal issue can be your missing link to health.

To remove metals safely, I recommend Coseva's Advanced TRS. TRS is a molecule that traps and contains heavy metals for easy removal by the body. It is tiny, so it gets into organs and deep to where metals are stored, and it's manufactured so it is 'empty' and ready to pick up metals from your body rather than bringing more into it.

You can purchase Advanced TRS at healthhomeandhappiness.com/trs or learn more on the Carnivore Resource Page.

Reason 5: Your expectations aren't realistic

We all love a good transformation story, but what we forget when we watch the 5-minute clip of someone losing 100 pounds in a year on the Carnivore diet is that it took a whole year!

If you feel like weight loss hasn't been fast enough, you should have more energy by now, or your muscles aren't growing big enough for your liking yet... you may need a good dose of patience!

The carnivore diet is a healing diet more than a weight loss diet, and sometimes that means you need to gain weight as your body gets the nutrients it needs to lose weight. If weight loss isn't what you're looking for, it may be that your body is doing deep healing as you provide it this excellent nutrition. If that is the case, you may feel more tired through this process.

With many deep healing protocols, it's common to get worse before you get better. This is called a herxheimer reaction, and it's because as the body heals, it stops covering up what is wrong, and goes into 'deep healing' mode. In the prescription-based medicine model, symptoms are often covered up rather than eliminated, but a herxheimer reaction can also be caused by antibiotics.

WHY DOES THE CARNIVORE DIET WORK?

Though simple and straightforward, the carnivore diet combines many healing principals into one easy-to-follow way of eating. Some things are avoided: Common allergens, oxalates, and nightshades. Some things are increased: Healthy fat, cholesterol, omega 3 fatty acids, and many other nutrients.

In doing the carnivore diet, we're able to balance the microbiome, stop autoimmune reactions, lose unneeded fat, increase insulin sensitivity, lower blood glucose levels, gain muscle and lean body mass, feed our brain, and more.

As with all dietary changes and meal plans, this is my opinion only, and I am not qualified to treat, prevent, or cure any disease.

Nutrient Density

When it comes to nutrient density of the nutrients we need to grow young children, repair and replace our own cells, and keep our body systems running, nothing can beat animal foods. Our stomachs are a ph of 1.5-3.5, which is very acidic and very good at getting the nutrients out of meat.

Consuming nose-to-tail (organ meat, not just muscle meat) helps boost the nutrient density.

Having a diet made up of easily absorbed, bio-available nutrients absolutely floods your body with the building blocks needed for it to do its own repair on everything from your brain to joints to muscles to blood cells.

Anti-Nutrients and Nutrient Absorption

Plant foods contain anti-nutrients, as well as nutrients. Animal foods have already had those anti-nutrients 'filtered out' when the animal ate the plants. With perfect digestion, balanced microbiome, and limited environmental toxins, it's likely that we are, as omnivores, able to easily deal with the anti-nutrients in plants and thrive on the good stuff that they provide. With an increased toxic load, generations of poor nutrition, and gut flora that is unbalanced, some of us have more trouble with anti-nutrients than others. Particularly, phytic acid that is found primarily in grains and legumes, is known to interfere with absorption of zinc, magnesium, calcium, and iron.

Anti-nutrients are not limited to phytic acid. Oxalates, lectins, phenols, and more are all found in plant foods, but not animal foods. This isn't to say that everyone should always avoid all plants, just be aware that there is a balance, and it will look different for everyone.

There is also evidence to suggest that these compounds, in a healthy person with a healthy digestive system, can provide 'resistance' that encourages the body to heal and strengthen. Think of carnivore as more of a resting and repairing protocol, and eating plants as pushing the body, or strength training. You wouldn't go into the gym and start an exercise program if you had two broken limbs and pneumonia... you'd rest while your body repaired itself. Then it may be time to introduce 'the gym' aka plants with anti-nutrients.

Oxalates are high in many plant foods and are correlated with decreased calcium absorption, kidney stones, and joint pain.

Lectins are found in approximately 30% of the plant food that the standard American eats including beans, grains, squash, and nightshades. Lectins are correlated with deterioration of the gut wall (leaky gut), autoimmune responses, and more.

Phenols and salicylates are found in brightly colored fruits and vegetables and can trigger autism and/or ADHD symptoms in some individual.

Sources:
https://www.ncbi.nlm.nih.gov/pmc/articles/PMC5983041/
https://www.ncbi.nlm.nih.gov/pubmed/26939264
https://www.ncbi.nlm.nih.gov/pubmed/15302522
https://www.ncbi.nlm.nih.gov/pubmed/24393738
https://feingold.org/

Allergies, Autoimmune, & Inflammation

These three are all tied to the body's overactive immune system. When we eat only animal products, avoiding any known allergies like dairy or eggs, the body gets a chance to calm down.

When we have leaky gut (see next page) it's likely that our body is reacting, or having an immune response, to every food we consume. Because all animal products are digested high up in the digestive system, the amount of nutrients that cross the lower gut and enter the bloodstream in undigested particles, triggers allergic, autoimmune, and inflammatory responses. These can include hives, rashes, joint pain, fatigue, swelling, diarrhea, and more.

Fiber & Digestion

Maybe one of the biggest myths of our time, fiber is actually bad for our digestion. Science shows over and over that when a no-fiber diet is consumed, digestion is improved! Studies of people with IBS, constipation, diarrhea, and other digestive issues all show either complete elimination or huge improvement when fiber is greatly reduced or eliminated.

When we don't eat stuff that we don't digest (fiber and other chemicals in plants) our body has to work so much less to digest our food. This gives our body a break to repair our gut and spend energy (along with the boost in nutrition) healing other parts of our body.

Sources:

https://www.ncbi.nlm.nih.gov/pmc/articles/PMC3435786/
https://www.ncbi.nlm.nih.gov/pmc/articles/PMC3544045/

Microbiome & Leaky Gut

Microbiome is big in the news now, and for good reason! This colony of microorganisms in our gut works together with our body to digest our food, line our gut wall to protect it, secrete enzymes, and even control our cravings! The microbiome is a big reason why it's hard to stop craving sugar even if we only have a little bit - if we eat sugar, we're feeding the bugs that also eat sugar.

And when we feed the bugs that eat sugar, they actually can 'poop' out chemicals that make their way into our bloodstream and up into our brain. Microorganisims are also survival of the fittest, so the ones that have this nifty adaptation (making us crave the foods they need) are the ones who survived. If you've ever felt like your brain was taken over and sugar cravings were beyond your control, you can blame your microbiome!

Thankfully when we stop eating sugar, wheat, or anything else that is unhealthy for us, those little bugs will die off. Usually this takes 72 hours, so don't be surprised if around the 3-day mark you get massive sugar cravings... and then after that they seem to disappear.

It's not just about the sugar and carb cravings, your microbiome can also send other signals to your brain causing fatigue, fuzzy thinking, and even psych issues like obsessive compulsive, depressive, or anxious thinking.

The bad bacteria, also called pathogenic bacteria, thrive on carbohydrates and reside low in the digestive tract. By going animal products only, or zero carb, the good bacteria take over and the bad are kept in check or completely eliminated. Your microbiome is always changing, due to the different foods you eat. When we avoid carbs, we speed up this change and quickly starve out the bad. Quick note: The microbiome is not all bad! We need a microbiome and the good bacteria in your gut that help

you digest food. The microbiome functions as a large part of your immune system, helps produce serotonin and dopamine (feel good hormones) and gives you cravings for the food that is good for you!

Sleep, Exercise, & Lean Body Mass

Good sleep is one of the biggest indicators of good health! Anecdotally, the carnivore diet is correlated with excellent quality sleep. With good sleep comes good energy during the day. Also anecdotally, but carnivore diet seems to go hand and hand with wanting to exercise.

We adapt an almost primitive mindset of enjoying fresh air, and active play - whether that's joining a coed sports team or running with the dog or playing with our kids. Flooded with the nutrients needed to repair and build muscles, it is common to have much more desire to exercise while on the carnivore diet. This weight bearing exercise increases lean body mass (muscles and bones) and improve metabolism. When the metabolism is running high not only is it easier to maintain a healthy weight, but a higher metabolism is also correlated with a general increase in overall health.

Insulin and Blood Glucose

Insulin resistance is a huge problem that affects the population. Most people take action in regards to insulin resistance when it causes weight gain. This often goes hand-in-hand with type 2 diabetes, though not always. Insulin resistance isn't a problem in only people who have type 2 diabetes or are overweight.

Insulin resistance is also linked with heart disease, cancer, infertility, and blood sugar fluctuations - getting light-headed or shaky between meals.

High blood glucose is a byproduct of insulin resistance. Type 1 diabetics have this as a result of not making enough (or any) insulin and requires insulin, though much less is required when eating low carb. Type 2 diabetics can lower their insulin resistance AND blood glucose by following a carnivore (or really any low carb diet).

If you have uncontrolled blood glucose (type 1 or 2) it is encouraged that you work with an endocrinologist as you transition onto keto or carnivore. There is a risk of ketoacidosis in those with uncontrolled blood sugar with the presence of ketones. Once the transition to low carb has been made, and blood glucose is under control, ketoacidosis is no longer a risk.

The carnivore diet stabilizes blood glucose because it is a very low carb diet, relying on ketones for energy rather than carbohydrates. This gives the body a break from needing to produce and respond to so much insulin, as the body gets energy directly from fat.

Sources:
https://www.ncbi.nlm.nih.gov/pmc/articles/PMC1204764/

Ketones and being in Ketosis

Ketosis is where most of the magic of carnivore comes from. When our body is running on fat, not carbs, we are providing our brain with ketones instead of glucose. Ketones have been extensively studied and are shown to help everything from neurological conditions including drug-resistant epilepsy and MS, addiction recovery, carb binges, anxiety and depression, and more.

To stay in ketosis on carnivore, some people have to keep their fat consumption around 80% calories from fat or more. But most of those who follow the carnivore diet will be in ketosis without tracking anything.

When searching medical journals for studies on ketosis, search 'very low carb diets' VLCD, modified atkins diets, and keto. The 'old version' of keto, used primarily as seizure control for the past century, also limited protein and liquids, which affected children's growth and the kidneys. Some doctors still recommend against 'keto' for this reason, they are looking at studies that restricted protein and liquids, on a protocol that was very hard to follow.

For more information about ketosis, check out the Keto Family Class, found on the Carnivore Resource Page.

WOMEN AND THE CARNIVORE DIET

Men: You are welcome (even encouraged!) to read here, but this section is for the ladies and specifics of the carnivore diet relating to periods, fertility, pregnancy, breastfeeding, birth control, social customs, and more.

We're going to have a frank discussion here, so please feel free to close the book if that bothers you. Unfortunately, how carnivore specifically relates to men isn't in my knowledge-field so there is no segment in this book just for the men. If you feel qualified to write one, please let me know and maybe I can include a guest writer for that chapter in future editions!

How does society react to women eating only meat?

Nobody will judge you for eating meat that wasn't already looking to judge you for something. You eating meat affects those around you 0%. The bias that women only eat light meals like salad or a piece of toast is fading. So many are feeling amazing on keto that they can't blame women for shunning carbs in favor of meat.

That said, we want to be careful to not over evangelize th carnivore diet and look for trouble where there is none. Because you're so easily satiated on the carnivore diet, and probably only eating 2-3 times a day, it's rare that people will even notice what you're eating.

The smile-nod-and change the subject approach works best for me. If someone comments that you're not eating any veggies, a quick 'nope' and 'so, how is your new puppy doing?' Subject change is the easiest way to do this. Remember, we're doing this for us, and we don't need to convert others in order to see results ourselves.

What about PMS? Why am I starving before my period?

When our hormones fluctuate through the month, our hunger naturally goes up right before our cycle starts.

Progesterone rises before your period starts, and it increases both your appetite. Serotonin dips, making you feel more irritable and tired.

When you're hungry, especially when it's linked to where you're at in your cycle, go ahead and eat! You may be intermittent fasting, or eating a certain number of calories a day for the rest of the month just fine.

If you feel unable to keep up with your appetite and cravings, my go-to recommendation is to brown up a pound of ground beef, salt it to taste and enjoy! If you still have cravings, and I know many of you aren't going to want to hear it, liver is a super food that squashes cravings! Saute some chicken liver in butter, sprinkle with salt, and enjoy!

How does the carnivore diet impact your cycle, sex drive, and fertility?

If you're not using birth control any more due to menopause or infertility, watch out! The carnivore diet is incredibly healing, anti-inflammatory, and can regulate hormones. Fertility returning on the carnivore diet even after years of going away is not unheard of.

If you chart your cycle and fertility signs, whether it's using the fertility awareness method as a form of birth control or just for your own personal knowledge, you will probably notice that your fertility signs are very strong while you're on carnivore! Around ovulation an increased sex drive, increased cervical mucus, and noticeable boost in mood and energy all point to increased fertility.

Yes, it's likely that your sex drive overall will increase. Healthy humans have healthy sex drives - it's just part of biology and the survival of the species.

No wonder there are so many adorable carnivore babies being born as the carnivore movement takes off!

As your hormones adjust, it is also common to have cycles become irregular before they become regular. If you are losing fat, especially if it's rapid, this can further mess with your cycle as we discuss next.

Candida (yeast) is commonly brought back into balance as part of the carnivore diet. Candida overgrowth is common among those who have been on multiple or strong courses of antibiotics, the birth control pill, or have been exposed to environmental toxins, and interferes with hormone balance, primarily responding to estrogen, progesterone, and producing seratonin. When Candida is brought back into balance, your hormones may take a bit to adjust as your body responds better to them.

Fat Loss & Whooshing

You may be doing the carnivore diet with your significant other, and notice that he is losing WAY faster than you are! Unfortunately this is common with women. We lose fat every day, but it tends to show up on the scale in starts and stops.

This rapid weight loss, and then nothing, and then a big drop again is called (totally scientific) *Whooshing*!

When we lose fat, our body takes the fat out of our fat cells and puts it into our blood, where it goes to our liver and is burned for energy. However, the body doesn't just take the fat out of the cells so they are deflated - it replaces the fat in the cell with water to 'hold' the cell in case we need to put more fat back in soon. After a few days, or even a few weeks, the body decides that those fat cells are unneeded for good, and it releases the water and the cell deflates.

When the cell deflates, we usually have to make a few trips to the bathroom that night to pee, and we get up the next morning and show a significant drop on the scale (even 2 lbs is quite significant - that's 8 sticks of butter!).

If you want to 'encourage' a whoosh, getting lots of rest and relaxation seems to help. I don't have any evidence of this, but I suspect that if our body is in stress mode, we often 'hold open' those fat cells with water until we're not stressed any more. The body is wired to survive, and making it easy to put fat back into a cell and save it for later is a survival technique. It's also common to get 'whooshes' around the time of ovulation, as the hormones adjust.

WEIGHT LOSS STALLS

Other than consuming too many calories (this will reveal itself when you calculate your calorie needs and weigh and measure all your food) there are other things that can cause weight loss stalling in women.

- Hormone fluctuations - our cycle encourages weight stalls, and even gains at certain times of the month. Embrace this, and know that you're 'banking' weight loss for other times of the month. This will change from individual to individual, but for most people our month's lowest weight will be the week before ovulation.
- Salt consumption! When we eat too much salt, our body will dilute it out with extra water. This, again causes bloating. Don't worry, it's just water weight. If you see the scale jump 2 lbs overnight this is most likely the cause. Remember, 2 lbs is ~ 7000 calories. It's unlikely that you EVER consume an excess 7000 calories, even if you do go off keto or binge on pork rinds with spinach dip.
- Exercise. When we start a new exercise program our muscles are tearing microscopically and then repairing themselves. Again, our body makes more blood and will send it to these muscles in need or repair and rebuilding. This causes a temporary (10ish days) increase in water weight. This is a good thing! Once those muscles have repaired and increased in size,

our metabolism will go up as muscle burns more, even at rest, than nothing or fat.

- You ate something you're allergic to. When we eat something that we are sensitive to, or allergic to, inflammation happens as our body tries to move it on out. This can cause us to hold onto water or 'bloat' up. If you know you're sensitive to certain foods, anticipate this reaction if you eat it!
- You went over your carbs. As we talked about, when you get into ketosis so your body takes the stored glycogen out of your muscles. With this glycogen comes the water that it is attached to - which provides a decent amount of bulk, and/or weight. *note! Your body will still 'spill ketones' in your urine even if you eat a high-carb meal. The brain and muscles prefer to run on glucose, so if you put sugar/carbs into your system, it will start feeding your brain and muscles glucose. This will cause the ketones already in your system to dump out. This is why you can have a 'cheat meal' and still show ketones in your urine if you are using the urine strips.

WEIGHT LOSS AND PERIOD PROBLEMS

When we burn lots of fat at once (as carnivore and keto lets us do), what is stored IN those fat cells along with the fat also becomes released. Namely, estrogen and toxins. If you feel like you're having a hormonal reaction (missed periods, heavy periods, acne) you can control this by slowing down your weight loss. That's right! All you need to do to slow down these symptoms is lose weight slower. This can be done by increasing your calories, but still keeping to carnivore foods.

Most women just deal with the hormone roller coaster and

are happy to get rid of the excess weight. Your mileage may vary, but this is a common 'carnivore symptom' that actually isn't attributed to carnivore at all - just that you lose weight efficiently on the carnivore diet.

THE CARNIVORE DIET AND CONFIDENCE IN WOMEN

You might not notice it at first, but as your body heals and becomes stronger, your sense of confidence will also bloom. This comes from thinking more clearly, more feel-good hormones being produced in a healthy gut, and even increased muscle mass. Yes, there is a correlation between increased core strength and self confidence!

Is it anger or passion?

Self confidence, in women especially, occasionally is mistaken as anger or arrogance. If think that you've suddenly become outspoken or angry on the carnivore diet, check in with yourself and see if this is actually increased self confidence and passion!

Passion gives our life great meaning and direction and is not to be discouraged. You can tell the difference between anger and passion because anger usually comes with a desire to harm, where passion comes with a desire to change for the overall good.

Index